Paddings and Strappings of the Foot

By

Charles Kaplan, D.P.M.
Peter D. Natale, D.P.M.
Terry L. Spilken, D.P.M.

Illustrator: **Howard A. Glaberman**

Futura Publishing Company
Mount Kisco, New York
1982

DEDICATION

We would like to dedicate this book to the memory of Emanuel E. Sugarman. Without his inspiration and effort, this book would never have become a reality.

FOREWORD

One of Man's most unique abilities through evolution is being able to walk on two feet. The necessity of now having to walk on hard concrete or asphalt surfaces without the give and take situation of soft dirt, sand, or grass, causes trauma to the foot, leg, and other structural entities. Since Man has become civilized, the evolutionary process of walking has been hindered in that Man now wears shoegear which might cause friction against some of the bony protuberances of the foot.

Some individuals have structural deformities of the foot and leg such as tibial torsion and hallux abducto valgus along with hammering of digits due to biomechanical forces. As we live longer more people develop circulatory problems such as peripheral vascular disease or arteriosclerosis obliterans, complicated with illnesses such as diabetes and decreased circulatory response to the distal aspects of the toes, which make a person prone to severe illnesses of the foot. In this day and age, if these problems are left unattended, it is quite possible that inflammation, infection, and even gangrene with amputation may occur in those people who are afflicted.

As a student of podiatry, I was greatly enlightened by the teaching of Dr. Emanuel Sugarman who continuously strived to make paddings and strappings that could be applied to our feet which would help people overcome their inadequacies in wearing foot gear and improve their biomechanical function. Through my work with Dr. Sugarman, at the New York College of Podiatric Medicine, I was able to learn many of his innovative techniques which have given many patients relief from their problems. Three of my students: Dr. Terry Spilken, Dr. Peter Natale, and Dr. Charles Kaplan have also seen a need to put together a written compendium on all the paddings and strappings which are used in the profession of podiatry. This fine publication is illustrated by Howard Glaberman, a student at the New York College of Podiatric Medicine.

I firmly believe this to be one of the first publications of its kind and expect that podiatrists, as well as students of podiatry, will find this book a necessity in the proper management of their podiatric patients. Many of the contributors of this book are also innovative men and women who are dedicated to the continuing ambulation of the public.

We feel that if we keep people walking in comfort, many of the degenerative illnesses which may afflict them in their geriatric years will be lessened. I greatly acknowledge and thank these aforementioned individuals for their work and wish to present this book to the students as well as to the practitioners of our great profession—Podiatry.

Bruce J. Frankel, D.P.M.

PREFACE

Padding—a pad can be any device or material used to supplement the body's own protective mechanisms.*

Shield—an appliance fashioned from some skin or fabric, applied for the purpose of relieving pressure or friction, or to protect a tender part upon the foot.**

Dressing—materials applied to a part for the purpose of excluding air or foreign substances, for stimulating repair and for protecting the affected area from external irritation.***

Strapping—a semi-rigid or elastic support that splints soft tissue and limits its function without completely immobilizing the part.*

It is our belief that a concise text covering the field of paddings and strappings for the foot has not been compiled. After an analysis of padding and strapping techniques and review of the literature dating back to the turn of the century, we have attempted to fill the missing void in the presentation of this material.

Each padding and strapping technique has been divided into the area of the foot it affects. These chapters cover the plantar, hallux, lesser toes, fifth digit, nails and heel. There are also introductory chapters on the theory behind these treatments and the various materials that can be used.

For the convenience of the reader, we also used a specific format for each pad or strapping technique. The indications for usage and the various materials needed are presented. Then the precise boundaries with instructions on the construction of these devices are described and are accompanied with drawings. Any final comments or additional instructions are given to complete the presentation.

We hope this guide to padding and strapping techniques will be used as a reference for podiatrists and help increase their skills in this field of therapy. We also hope this book will be of value as a guide to the student or assistant in learning this important aspect of conservative therapy.

We wish to gratefully acknowledge the contributions made by those practitioners whose works are included in this volume. It is hoped that their dedication and their inventiveness serve as inspirational models for all of us who endeavor to relieve the maladies that afflict the human foot.

---

*Hlavac: *The Foot Book.*
**Burnett and Gross: *Practice of Podiatry.*
***Gross: *Modern Foot Therapy.*

CONTRIBUTORS

Lester Bluhm, D.P.M.
Past President, Podiatry Society, State of New York
Past President, Academy of Podiatric Medicine

Philip R. Brachman, D.P.M.
President Emeritus, Dr. William M. Scholl College of Podiatric Medicine
Past President, Illinois Podiatry Association

Joseph C. D'Amico, D.P.M., F.A.C.F.O., F.A.C.P.
Professor and Chairman, Division of Orthopedic Sciences, New York College
   of Podiatric Medicine

Murray Edelstein, D.P.M.
Diplomate, American Board of Podiatric Surgery
Past President, New York College of Podiatric Medicine

Bruce J. Frankel, D.P.M.
Associate Director and Professor, Department of Basic Operative Podiatry,
   New York College of Podiatric Medicine
Director, Podiatry Residency Program of Brooklyn

Irwin Hanover, D.P.M.
Editor-in-Chief, *Current Podiatry*

Leonard Hymes, D.P.M.
Past President, American Academy of Podiatry Administration
Professor of Podiatry, Pennsylvania College of Podiatric Medicine

Robert R. Krout, D.P.M.
Member, Podiatric Circulatory Society

Raymond K. Locke, D.P.M., F.A.C.F.S.
Adjunct Clinical Instructor, Illinois College of Podiatric Medicine
Associate Clinical Professor, California College of Podiatric Medicine (at Los
   Angeles County Hospital, University of Southern California Medical Center)

Elizabeth H. Roberts, D.P.M.
Professor Emeritus, New York College of Podiatric Medicine
Former Chairperson, New York State Board for Podiatry

Ralph E. Sansone, D.P.M., D.S.C., F.A.C.F.R., F.A.C.P.M.
Past President, Connecticut Podiatry Society
Past President, American College of Foot Roentgenologist
Past President, American College of Podiatric Medicine

Richard O. Schuster, D.P.M., F.A.C.F.O., A.B.P.O.
Past President, American College of Foot Orthopedists
Past President, American Society of Podiatric Medicine
Past President, American Board of Podiatric Orthopedists

Emanuel E. Sugarman, D.P.M.*
Chairman and Professor, Department of Basic Operative Podiatry, New York
    College of Podiatric Medicine

---

*Deceased.

TABLE OF CONTENTS

I

THEORY

PRELIMINARY CONSIDERATIONS

For padding or strapping techniques to give optimum results, one must understand the mechanisms involved in how feet function. This implies not only a knowledge of the anatomy of the foot and leg but also an understanding of the mechanics of movement. Biomechanics will explain why many of the pathologic conditions exist and the correct areas where the strain, pressure or friction should be relieved. The correct therapy must be instituted to prevent the progressive development of foot disease. A treatment plan should always take into consideration the health, age and attitude of the patient. The patient must approve and cooperate with the therapy about to be undertaken.

PRINCIPLES

There are numerous principles that should be followed for padding and strapping to be effective. No matter how scientific the construction, if these principles are not considered, the results might be more annoying to the patient than the

This section incorporates the theory and practice of Doctors Murray Edelstein, Bruce Frankel, Elizabeth Roberts, and Richard Schuster.

original complaint. The following principles are essential to the comfort of the patient.

1. The correct thickness of the pad must be used. A pad which is too thin will not accomplish its primary function. A pad too thick could cause considerable pain and discomfort. This could cause constriction or pressure between the shoe and the foot.

2. The correct size and shape of the material must be used. This is dependent on the exact location and type of function that is desired. If the size or shape is not correctly measured, the symptoms might not be relieved and the possibility exists that more discomfort might ensue. No part of the material should impinge upon any area of irritation or inflammation.

3. If an aperture is necessary, it must have the proper shape. Too small an opening can put pressure directly into the area from which one wants to alleviate the forces. Too big an aperture means that normal weight bearing or pressure will exist. Apertures should be circular or oval and just slightly larger than the lesion.

4. The pads must be properly skived so pressure is evenly distributed and high points avoided.

Pressure must be distributed away from the area being protected and a correctly skived pad will accomplish this.

5. The pad must be put on the skin in the correct manner, utilizing adherents when necessary. This could avoid slippage and possible irritation from the pad applied.

6. The pad should be covered so that there are no free edges. This prevents a free edge from being raised from the skin. This edge might then be caught by the hosiery or shoe and its position disturbed. Adhesive plaster, moleskin, lamb's wool and self-adhering gauze are examples of materials to accomplish this function. More information can be obtained in the Materials chapter of this book.

7. The ends of the material should be cut round. This helps prevent loosening of the corners which is a common finding with sharp edges.

8. In most cases, padding should be built up proximal to the lesion or area to be protected.

9. Strappings should be applied with the correct amount of pressure. Too tight and the circulation might be constricted and necessary expansion of the tissues prevented. Too loose and no therapeutic effects will be gained. A strapping that completely encircles a toe might compromise the circulation to that part.

10. The skin should not be puckered or pulled into folds by excessive tension. Air gaps should not be left between the material and the skin.

11. Joints should not be inadvertently immobilized. Undesired restriction of a joint's range of motion might ensue needlessly and cause added problems.

12. When using skin adherents, never apply them onto the lesion itself. Always permit the adherent to dry thoroughly before applying the pad.

13. Paraffin applied over the finished pad or tape will prevent the material from sticking to the stockings or shoes. It will also give the material some degree of resistance to water.

GENERAL PURPOSES

1. relief from pain
2. to improve foot function
3. to lessen trauma to sensitive areas
4. to compensate for an imbalance
5. to afford a better treading surface
6. to increase the support or protection of symptomatic areas
7. to reduce the trauma of weight bearing
8. to reduce bony subluxations
9. to eliminate excrescences
10. to protect areas from friction, pressure and shearing forces
11. to allow ambulation for postoperative patients
12. to keep digits in the correct postsurgical position

SPECIFIC PURPOSES*

1. to protect
   a. areas of pain and inflammation
   b. areas after surgery
   c. where there is pressure from weight bearing, from shoes or from another part of the foot
   d. where there is friction
   e. where there is rigidity
2. to deflect
   a. pressure away from painful areas
   b. through equalization of weight bearing by redistribution of the weight
3. to correct
   a. hypermobility
   b. an incipient deformity and weakness
   c. lack of muscle tone
   d. overstrain of muscles
   e. overstrain of ligaments
   f. overstrain of fascia

COMPLICATIONS

Potential problems can develop with the incorrect use of padding and strapping techniques. The following can be the cause of failure of one of these modes of treatment.

1. Incorrect size or shape of material used. This will defeat the purpose of a well planned therapy. Each padding or strapping should remain in the correct boundaries as described for each technique. Plantar pads should cover as much area

as possible to distribute weight bearing and avoid concentrations in one particular area.

2. Incorrect density—either too firm or too soft to accomplish any correction. Too much bulk could cause pressure of the shoe against the foot.

3. Incorrect placement on the foot or leg of correctly cut material. The therapy is of no value unless it is positioned over the correct anatomical area. Otherwise, nearby tissues (such as an adjacent toe) could cause irritation of that part.

4. Patients who cannot tolerate the pad or strap designed—some patients cannot tolerate certain therapies even when they are correctly prepared. Other treatments with the same purposes should then be incorporated. When a treatment cannot be tolerated by the patient, another one accomplishing the same goal can be substituted.

5. Function may not be improved with the use of the therapy selected. Reevaluation of the problem is then necessary to find another treatment that will work to improve the function desired.

6. The type of shoegear and its usage may not allow the pad or strap designed to function. It is essential to evaluate the type of shoegear your patient will be using. Some of the therapies are negated by certain footgear. The shoe might alter the biomechanics and functioning of the limb and this must be considered before a suc-

*Alan Challoner in *British Journal of Chiropody*, 1964.

cessful therapy can be instituted.

7. The patient's chief complaint may have been remedied but a new problem has been created. By altering one incorrect attitude for another incorrect one will just create a strain on another part of the anatomy. The primary purpose of padding and strapping techniques should be to render the patient asymptomatic. One does not want to alleviate one problem by creating a new one.

8. Patients may have allergies to the materials used and develop a contact dermatitis. Another problem may be maceration and a breakdown of the skin under the material.

SKIVING

Skiving is "a process by which the edges of a shield are thinned or bevelled to a feather edge." The principal reasons for skiving are as follows:

1. Unnecessary pressure is avoided. Excessive thickness of a pad could create areas of friction where the pad meets the skin.

2. Skived edges will allow the pad to better adhere to the skin and form a better contour with the body.

3. Skived edges will allow the reinforcement shielding (binder) to better adhere over the pad and make closer contact with the skin without leaving any gaps or openings.

4. An aperture should be skived to avoid irritation to the tissues directly under the tender area.

5. To provide the least amount of bulk.

SKIVING TECHNIQUES

1. Cut the material to the correct size and shape desired.

2. Hold material on a smooth piece of glass, wood or stone with the non-cutting hand.

3. Hold the skiving knife in the cutting hand and cut away from yourself with an oblique stroke. The effect of this motion is to create a bevelled edge.

4. Cut the edges of the pad and thin them to a feathered edge.

5. Obtain a uniform thickness around the periphery and maintain a smooth surface.

6. Make certain the entire surface of the pad is uniformly smooth.

CUTTING TECHNIQUES

1. The scissor should be held on the thumb and fourth finger.
2. Wax on the scissors will facilitate cutting of the material.
3. Always remove the plastic backing on adhesive material before cutting.
4. Fold the material so the sticky side is out when rounding edges to make a symmetrical cut.
5. Try to always use the heel of the scissors when cutting material.
6. When using curved scissors, use the convex part.

II
BINDINGS

INTRODUCTION

After a pad has been placed in the correct position, it is very important to cover the finished product. A binding or dressing not only excludes air and foreign substances but also maintains the correct position of the shield applied. The lesion should be protected with any medication desired by the practitioner. An opening over a lesion (e.g., aperture, horseshoe) should then be covered with a small piece of cotton or gauze. The binding of tape, elastoplast or any other desired material can then be applied.

Contained in this chapter are some basic approaches used to secure paddings in place. Adhesive strips, elastoplast or coban are very common adaptations applied over the shield after a skin adherent is used. The edges of all bindings should be rounded to secure the proper fit.

OVAL BINDINGS

INDICATIONS

Binds down any padding of an oval shape.

MATERIALS

Adhesive tape, elastoplast or any other desired material.

BOUNDARIES

Covers paddings on toes, plantar, dorsum, hallux, etc. The binding extends slightly over the boundaries of the pad to be covered.

CONSTRUCTION

1. Cut a piece of desired material slightly larger on all sides than the pad to be covered.
2. Adhere the binding over the pad onto the skin after applying an appropriate skin adherent.

ADDITIONAL COMMENTS

1. ⅛" adhesive strips may be used to anchor this binding in place.
2. Elastoplast used on a toe should stretch along the axis of that toe so that it flexes with the toe.

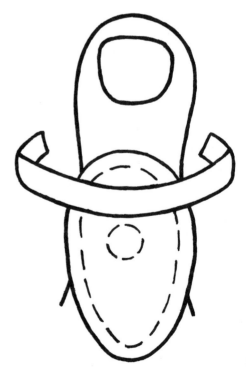

Figure 1. Oval Binding

IRON CROSS

INDICATIONS

To bind down paddings or strappings at the distal aspect of any toe or the area of the heel.

MATERIALS

For a toe, a strip of 1″ adhesive tape by 1½″-2″ long. For a heel, a strip of 3″ or 4″ adhesive tape by 1½″-2″ long.

BOUNDARIES

Covers the distal aspect of the toe to the distal interphalangeal joint. Covers the entire surface of the heel from medial to lateral, anterior and posterior.

CONSTRUCTION

1. From each of the four corners make a diagonal cut toward the center. Extend the cut about half-way to the center (Fig. 1).
2. Place the uncut center of the tape on the distal most aspect of the toe or the center of the heel (Fig. 2).
3. Smooth down the dorsal and plantar wings.
4. Smooth down the medial and lateral wings. Mild tension while applying these edges will avoid any overlap.

ADDITIONAL COMMENTS

On a toe, an anchor may be beneficial by using a ⅛″ × 2″ strip of adhesive tape.

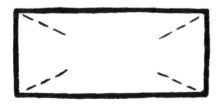

Figure 1.

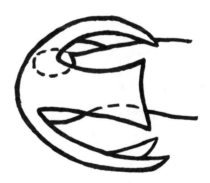

Figure 2.

SELF-ADHERING GAUZE BINDINGS AND LAMB'S WOOL

INDICATIONS

To bind down paddings by wrapping material over the shield.

MATERIALS

Self-adhering gauze bindings in various widths and lengths and/or lamb's wool.

BOUNDARIES

Covers the pad with strips of material that adheres to itself.

CONSTRUCTION

1. Wrap the gauze around the padding and allow it to adhere to itself (Fig. 1).
2. Completely cover the pad with the gauze. End the material between the toes.

ADDITIONAL COMMENTS

1. These materials have a tendency to self-tighten when being unrolled. Loosen material first and then apply it to the foot.
2. Distal aspects of toes can be covered by folding the material back upon itself (Fig. 2).
3. The same binding can be accomplished with the use of lamb's wool. First apply a skin adherent to the toe and pad. Apply the lamb's wool and cover the entire area with rubber cement or collodion.
4. Powder with talc all finished products.
5. Remember not to make the binding too thick in any area.

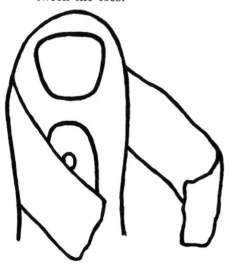

Figure 1.

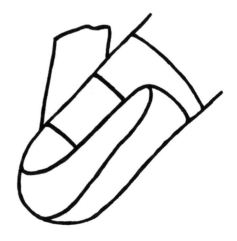

Figure 2.

T-STRAPS

INDICATIONS
To bind down any padding used in the area of a toe.

MATERIALS
Usually made out of elastoplast but adhesive tape may be used.

BOUNDARIES
The broad part of the cover extends over the pad and the straps go through the interspace.

CONSTRUCTION
1. Cut a 1″ square of material or larger if necessary.
2. Fold the material in half with the sticky side out.
3. Make a ¼″ cut about ⅛″ from one corner. Turn the scissors 90° to the longer side of the pad. Cut straight and round the edge. The cover being made should be approximately ½″ wide.
4. Adhere the bottom of the T over the pad to be covered. Use the straps of the T to bind the cover through the interspace.

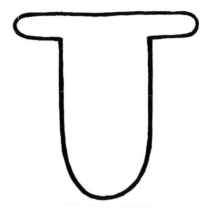

Figure 1. T-Strap

ADDITIONAL COMMENTS
1. Always be sure the top of the T is not too wide. This might cause irritation in the interspace.
2. This basic shape can be used on other parts of the foot. A common place is on the heel. The flap extends over the plantar of the heel and the strips cover the medial and lateral sides of the ankle.

FIGURE EIGHT ANCHOR STRIP

INDICATIONS

To bind down any corrective paddings used on a digit. Modifications can be made to bind larger pads on other parts of the foot.

MATERIALS

⅛" wide strip of adhesive tape approximately 6" in length.

BOUNDARIES

This binding will extend from the distal aspect of the pad and end just proximal to the proximal end of the pad.

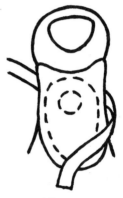

Figure 1.

CONSTRUCTION

1. Place one end of the adhesive strip just proximal to the pad on the dorsomedial aspect (Fig. 1).
2. Run the strip on a diagonal towards the distal lateral aspect. Bring the piece around the toe on the plantar aspect from lateral to medial. Come across the dorsum, thus securing the distal aspect of the pad (Fig. 2).
3. Return the strip to the plantar aspect on the lateral side. Run the strip on a diagonal to the medial side of the toe. Return to the dorsum and continue on a diagonal to the lateral proximal side of the toe (Fig. 3).

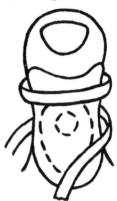

Figure 2.

ADDITIONAL COMMENTS

1. If the binding is too tight it will impede the circulation.
2. Do not cover an aperture with any of the strips.

Figure 3.

TUBULAR GAUZE BINDINGS

INDICATIONS
To bind a padding on a toe or to hold a dressing in position.

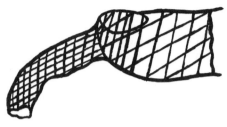

MATERIALS
Tubular gauze (usually No. 1 for a digit and No. 2A for the hallux) and ⅛" adhesive tape or self-adhering gauze.

Figure 1.

BOUNDARIES
Covers the entire toe from its distal aspect to the sulcus.

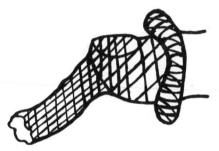

CONSTRUCTION
1. Using a piece of tubular gauze approximately 3"-4" long, place half of it over your own finger (Fig. 1).
2. Roll the material back on itself so half of the piece is now rolled (Fig. 2).

Figure 2.

3. Take the gauze off your finger and place the rolled edge at the distal end of the digit.
4. Unroll the gauze onto the toe so that half is on the toe and the other half free (Fig. 3).

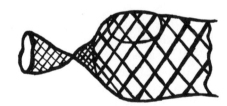

5. Twist the free end for one complete turn (180°). Slide the free end over the toe (Fig. 4).

Figure 3.

6. Secure an anchor around the free edges near the sulcus. ⅛" adhesive felt or self-adhering gauze work very well as the material for the anchor.

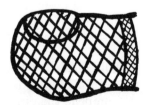

Figure 4.

ADDITIONAL COMMENTS

1. Some brands of tubular gauze include an applicator to apply this binding. Instructions on the use of the applicator are included with the material.

2. Do not allow excess material to collect in the interspace or sulcus which might irritate the skin.

III

MATERIALS

Adhesive Tape
Dental Cotton Roll
Elastoplast
Felt
Adhesive Felt
Foam Rubber
Adhesive Foam
Lamb's Wool
Moleskin
Moldable Silicone Gels

Hypoallergenic Tape
Self-Adhering Gauze
Sponge Rubber
Tubular Foam
Tubular Gauze
Latex
Latex Techniques
The Construction of Latex
   Appliances

INTRODUCTION

There are numerous types of material available for the construction of the various pads, shields and straps described in this text. Each material has specific properties that make their use more valuable under certain conditions. The compressibility, resilience and durability of each material should be considered before its usage. What will follow is a summary of the basic materials being used. It is not an attempt at describing every material that could be used. Each practitioner can experiment with various materials until the properties required are found.

ADHESIVE TAPE

This comes on rolls in widths from one-eighth inch to three inches. Its use is primarily for securing other material to the foot and as the medium for strapping. The tape in widths of one-eighth and one-quarter of an inch is particularly useful in the region of the toes.

DENTAL COTTON ROLL

It comes in three and six-inch lengths and one-quarter inch width, generally in bundles of fifty. Its primary use is in the fabrication of crest pads filling the space in the web of the toes (the sulcus).

ELASTOPLAST

Elastoplast comes in rolls in widths from one to three inches. This is a stretchable self-adhering tape that can apply compression as well as securing a padding to an area. It can be used on people who have a hypersensitivity to adhesive tape.

FELT

Felt comes in thicknesses ranging from one-sixteenth of an inch to one inch in width. It is generally composed of a combination of wool and cotton which affects the degree of firmness. The thinnest felts are used for work around the toes. The thicker material works well on the plantar and dorsal aspects. This material can be adhered to the skin or in the shoe with a skin adherent or a rubber cement. All pads made of felt must be skived to a feather edge. Felt made of all wool has fairly good resistance to compression and has immediate complete recovery. Felt with part wool and cotton is fairly easily compressed but has a slow but complete recovery.

ADHESIVE FELT

This is the same felt as described above with an adhesive backing protected by an easily removable plastic. The need for an adherent is avoided.

FOAM RUBBER

Foam rubber comes in thicknesses ranging from one-sixteenth inch to one inch in width and can usually be obtained in three densities: soft, medium, and firm. It is composed of a series of interconnecting air cells thus allowing it to breathe when next to the skin. It is therefore cooler than sponge rubber. It is very easily compressed with a reasonable but complete recovery.

ADHESIVE FOAM

This is the same foam as above with an adhesive backing protected by an easily removable plastic. The need for an adherent is avoided.

LAMB'S WOOL

Lamb's wool comes in long fibers in bulk packaging. It can be used to separate toes, as insoles in shoes, and to bind down pads when adhesive tape is contraindicated. The material is bound to itself with the use of rubber cement, flexible collodion, or clear nail polish. It is seldom adhered to the skin itself.

MOLESKIN

Moleskin comes in rolls from one to ten yards long and from three to twelve inches wide. It has an adhesive backing with an easily removable plastic. The need for an adherent is avoided. It is a very thin material, approximately one-sixteenth of an inch, that does not stretch nor pull out of shape while on the skin. It is also very pliable and soft, thus avoiding the necessity for skiving. Its primary use is as a protection over slightly irritated skin after debridement.

MOLDABLE SILICONE GELS

This product usually contains silicone or similar chemical and a catalyst. Instructions are given to mix the two ingredients and a moldable product is formed that will harden in a short period of time. The doctor can now hand-fabricate numerous shapes and forms to meet the needs of the individual patient. This type of padding is removable and reusable for the patient and easily cleaned with either alcohol or soap and water. The material should have a high degree of tear strength and be hydrophobic (resistant to water damage). Its usage is as heloma durum and molle pads, crests for toes, tailor's bunion shields, postoperative splints, hallux valgus shields, exostosis shields, toe splints, protection for club nails, correction for over- or underlapping toes and as attachments to other fabricated devices. Its main advantage is the ease of fabrication.

HYPOALLERGENIC TAPE

This tape comes in rolls in widths from one-half to three inches. This type of tape was designed to hold securely with minimal irritation to the skin and with ease of removal. It is generally microporous allowing air to reach the skin and discouraging bacterial growth and maceration. It is mainly used on diabetics and persons known to be hypersensitive to adhesive tape.

SELF-ADHERING GAUZE

This comes on rolls in widths from one-half inch to three inches. This material does not adhere to skin, hair, clothing or other materials. This material only adheres to itself. Water does not affect the binding capability of this gauze. It is used primarily when adhesive tape is contraindicated for binding down other materials.

SPONGE RUBBER

Sponge rubber comes in sheets ranging from one-sixteenth to three-quarters of an inch. It can be used in soft, medium or firm densities. It is composed of chemically blown cells of either nitrogen or normal air. It is not a breathable material next to the skin and is therefore not as cool as foam rubber. It contains more rubber per square inch than foam. It has fairly good resistance to compression with an immediate and complete recovery.

TUBULAR FOAM

This foam comes in tubes twelve inches in length, in widths of small, medium and large. It is easily slipped over a toe or hallux and

usage is primarily as a removable pad. The foam material acts as a protection over an excrescence in these areas. It has the same basic properties as foam rubber.

TUBULAR GAUZE

This is a seamless gauze that comes in a tubular form. It is obtainable in various sizes. The most popular for podiatric uses are sizes 1 (⅝"), 2 (⅞"), 2A (1⅛"), and 3 (1½"). It conforms to the contours of the toes or foot when applied. It is primarily used as a binder when adhesive tape is contraindicated. Sizes 1 and 2 are primarily used on the lesser toes while size 2A is used on the hallux. This gauze is a stretchable material that can be applied with a special applicator available from the manufacturer.

LATEX

Latex (crude natural rubber) is a milk-white, slightly viscous fluid that is obtained from the rubber tree by draining incisions that have been cut into the bark. It has the unique capacity to solidify to a durable, flexible polymer upon exposure to air and its utilization in many industries, as well as its application in podiatry, rests upon this property.

The latex commonly used in podiatry appliance fabrication has certain chemical additives that modify the polymerization reaction, slowing it to a workable rate. For best results, liquid latex should be stored in a dark, tightly covered glass jar. Use latex from a podiatry supply house because plain latex sticks to itself after hardening.

THE LATEX TECHNIQUE

The latex technique can be utilized to construct appliances that are indicated in the management of a wide variety of pedal conditions and lesions. Common applications of these devices include the treatment of hallux abducto valgus, hammer digit syndrome, "Tailor's bunion," various pedal ulcerations and forefoot conditions. Other entities, some quite specialized, have been treated with the use of latex, or latex-coated, appliances.

In general, this technique seems to be particularly well suited to the management of rigid foot deformities and chronic conditions, rather than in cases of flexible deformities or acute conditions. When shields that are more durable and permanent are required, or when the adherance of a shield to the skin of the patient is contraindicated, latex devices can be utilized to great advantage, since their thickness, general contour, and cushioning ability remain relatively constant over a period of many months.

In certain instances, latex appliances are not useful and, in fact, may be contraindicated. Cases of uncontrollable hyperhydrosis or hypersensitivity to latex, for example, as well as factors such as patient compliance, cost, or the occupation of the patient (petroleum products are deleterious to latex) can prevent the use and/or effectiveness of these devices.

In the final analysis, the experience of numerous podiatric practitioners has demonstrated that latex therapy can be a highly successful modality in the treatment of many podiatric conditions.

THE CONSTRUCTION OF LATEX APPLIANCES

The construction of latex appliances entails basically two distinct processes: casting, wherein one obtains an accurate model of the foot-part to be treated, and shield fabrication, wherein one applies successive coats of liquid latex to the casted foot-part and incorporates the necessary shielding components. Each process must be carefully completed, in a given sequence of steps, so that the desired product can be obtained.

Casting

The plaster-strip method is the most commonly utilized technique (Polokoff, 1939). Other less commonly used methods have been proposed (Vosburg, 1937; Meldman, 1940).

A. Materials (plaster-strip technique): indelible marking pen, skin lubricant (petroleum jelly, mineral oil), 1-inch wide plaster strips (6 to 8 inches in length), wooden applicator stick, separating medium (tincture of green soap, liquid glass), powdered plaster.

B. Technique
   1. Using accepted methods, re-

duce the excrescence with a sanding disc.

2. Trim the nails reasonably short.
3. Mark the lesion with indelible material.
4. Moisten the entire area to be casted with a skin lubricant; lesser toe casts should extend at least 3 inches proximal to the lesion; hallux and 5th toe casts should extend at least 4 inches proximal to the lesion.
5. Dip the plaster strips in water; remove only the excess liquid.
6. Apply 4 to 6 layers of the plaster strips to the area, in a direction that is parallel to the long axis of the digits; do not encircle the toes; "work" the plaster into the interdigital spaces with a probe or wooden applicator stick.
7. Wait 3 to 5 minutes for the plaster to set.
8. Remove the cast from the foot by gently working the plaster away from the skin surfaces and pulling it off in the direction in which the toes curve.
9. Let the cast dry thoroughly, overnight if possible.
10. Pour a separating medium into the negative mold ensuring that all surfaces are well coated.
11. Puncture pin holes in the distal end of the toe cast (to discourage formation of air pockets when positive casting material is poured).

12. Mix positive casting material to a sour cream consistency in a mixing bowl.
13. Pour positive casting material into the negative mold, at a constant flow rate so as to minimize the formation of air pockets.
14. Following manufacturers directions, allow sufficient time for the positive casting material to harden.
15. Place entire filled negative mold in water for 5 minutes.
16. Remove negative mold from positive cast by peeling plaster strips away.
17. Darken (or remark) indelible transfer outlines on the positive cast.
18. Sand positive cast smooth while retaining all essential contours.

Additional Comments (from various sources): Fill minor defects in the positive cast with plaster or wax. Make a razor cut in the back of the negative mold to facilitate removing it from around the hardened positive cast. Before the positive casting material hardens, embed a firm wire, wooden applicator stick, or similar item into the material; alternatively, screw a wall-hook, eye-hook, or cup-hook into the hardened positive to facilitate the dipping process. Fashion a plaster stand in which to place the positive cast during the drying periods of the layering process; the wire or wooden applicator stick can be positioned into this.

Shield Fabrication

A. Materials—liquid latex, hot air blower; felt, sponge rubber, chamois, or moleskin of suitable thicknesses; rubber cement, scissors, powder.

B. Technique
   1. Dip the prepared positive cast into the liquid latex for several seconds until all exposed areas of the plaster cast are coated; position the cast to allow for air drying, either hanging it from an embedded hook or placing it upright into a plaster stand (see *Additional Comments* above).
   2. Allow at least 30 minutes for drying; this time may be hastened by the use of a hot air blower.
   3. Repeat the dipping-drying sequence 1 to 5 additional times.
   4. Fashion a suitable pad, shield, or build-up that will when positioned offer protection to the lesion being treated; use appropriate materials, of suitable thicknesses, and follow the principles that have been established for the proper design of shields.
   5. Position the pad, shield, or build-up in the proper position on the positive latex-layered cast and adhere it in place with rubber cement.
   6. Repeat the dipping-drying sequence 3 to 12 additional times, depending on the wear anticipated.
   7. Allow the final latex coat to dry 24 to 48 hours.
   8. Remove the device from the positive cast carefully; trim the device, rounding all edges and paying attention to portions of the finished product that will fit in interdigital or web areas.
   9. Powder the device and dispense to the patient; instruct the patient to powder the device each day before wearing.

Additional Comments (from various sources): Cut out the toenail area of the latex device to help avoid tearing the product and to aid in ventilation. Perforate the device with multiple small holes to aid in ventilation; this is especially important in hot weather areas. Incorporate soft linings into latex devices for dermatitis or other sensitive patients. This can be accomplished by either adhering thin felt, moleskin, or chamois into the finished device or by applying these materials directly to the positive cast (soft surface contacting the cast surface) before the latex coats are applied.

REFERENCES

Polokoff, M.M., *Clinical Journal of Chiropody, Podiatry and Pedic Surgery*, 10 (6): 189, 1939.

Vosburg, G.B., *Clinical Journal of Chiropody, Podiatry and Pedic Surgery*, 9 (7): 249, 1937.

Meldman, E.C., *Chiropody Record*, 23 (7): 151, 1940.

Strahs, R., *Clinical Journal of Chiropody, Podiatry and Pedic Surgery*, 11 (2): 54, 1940.

Dietz, L.H., *Clinical Journal of Chiropody, Podiatry and Pedic Surgery*, 12 (2): 63, 1941.

Batts, V.L., Balloqui, P.E., *The Chiropodist*, 12 (5): 348, 1950.

Moon, C.L., *Current Chiropody*, 2 (11): 9, 1953.

Block, I.H., *Current Chiropody*, 5 (9): 9, 1956.

IV

PLANTAR

THE PLANTAR ACCOMMODATIVE PAD

INDICATIONS

To disperse weight away from painful lesions occurring at any one of the four lesser metatarsal heads.

MATERIALS

1. ¼" adhesive felt.
2. Spray adhesive.
3. Soft lead pencil.
4. Skiving knife.

BOUNDARIES

The pad will extend just beyond the metatarsal parabola distally, the lateral side will extend flush with the lateral border of the foot. The medial side will follow the first metatarsal shaft proximally then curve superiorly to the talonavicular articulation. The posterior aspect of the pad will cross the foot just anterior to the calcaneal tuberosity.

CONSTRUCTION

1. Cut a piece of ¼" adhesive felt into a 7" × 4" rectangle.
2. Lightly adhere the pad to the foot so that one 7" edge lies flush with the lateral aspect of the foot. The posterior edge of

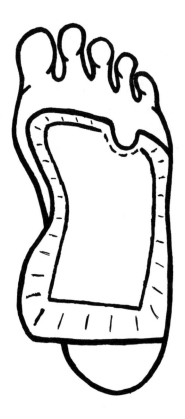

Berger, O.R.: Orthopedic padding. *Chiropody Record*, 26 (7): 1943, pp. 135-139.

the pad should rest just distal to the weight-bearing tuberosity of the calcaneus.

3. By palpation locate the head of the fifth metatarsal and, with a soft pencil, mark the pad so that you follow the metatarsal

parabola to the first metatarsal head. Make sure that this pencil line falls just distal to the parabola created by the metatarsal heads.

4. The outline of the pad is continued with the marker along the medial inferior border of the first metatarsal shaft and continues to the first metatarsal cuneiform articulation and superiorly to the talonavicular articulation. The line continues abruptly inferior to the medial inferior border of the heel at the back of the pad.

5. The pad is now skived to a thin edge on all sides except at the metatarsal parabola where the skive should be more abrupt.

6. The lesion to be treated is now marked and transferred to the adhesive felt.

7. Cut an aperture from the felt pad that will approximate the size of the lesion.

8. Apply spray adhesive to the plantar aspect of the foot and adhere the finished pad.

ADDITIONAL COMMENTS

The pad can be easily secured for longer wear by adhering strips of one-inch adhesive tape across the plantar aspect of the foot at various points.

MORTON'S COMPENSATING PAD

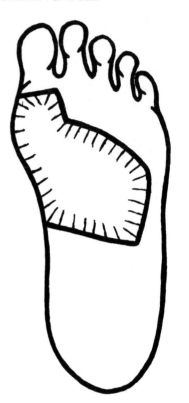

INDICATIONS
For symptomatic congenital short first metatarsal with a painful lesion under the second metatarsal head.

MATERIALS
1. ¼" adhesive felt.
2. Soft lead marking pencil.

BOUNDARIES
The pad will extend distally on the medial side of the foot to fall approximately ¼" distal to the first metatarsal head. The remaining anterior border will fall just proximal to the metatarsal heads. The posterior aspect of the pad will cross the foot at the first metatarsal cuneiform articulation.

CONSTRUCTION
1. Cut a piece of ¼" felt into approximately a 3" × 4" rectangle.
2. Place the pad on the foot so that it covers all the metatarsal heads and is flush with the medial and lateral sides of the foot.
3. With a soft lead pencil draw a line from just behind the fifth metatarsal head diagonally across the foot just behind the metatarsal heads to a point between the first and second meta-

tarsal heads. From here the line continues distally between the first and second metatarsal heads to a point at the distal aspect of the first metatarsal head. The line is then carried in a medial direction to the medial border of the first metatarsal. The line then passes proximally following the contour of the first metatarsal shaft and changes direction to cross the foot in a lateral direction at the first metatarsal cuneiform ar-

Berger, O.R.: Orthopedic padding. *Chiropody Record*, 26 (7): 1943, pp. 111-112.

ticulation. The line is finished by continuing to the starting point by following the lateral border of the fifth metatarsal shaft proximally.

4. The pad is now skived according to the following specifications. The extension under the hallux is skived leaving ⅛" anteriorly. The front end of the extension should be finished with a rounded skive. The front of the pad behind the four lesser metatarsal heads should receive an abrupt skive. Do not skive the pad at the second metatarsal head. Here maximum thickness is needed for protection. The medial and lateral sides of the pad receive sharp skives being somewhat longer posteriorly than anteriorly. The posterior skive should begin approximately midshaft of the first metatarsal.

5. Spray the plantar aspect of the foot with adhesive and adhere in place. The lateral posterior corner of the extension is placed as closely around the second metatarsal head as possible without putting additional pressure on it.

ADDITIONAL COMMENTS

The pad can be easily secured for longer wear by adhering strips of 1" adhesive tape across the plantar aspect of the foot at various points.

PAD FOR DORSAL HYPERMOBILITY OF THE FIRST SEGMENT

INDICATIONS
To control motion in a hypermobile first ray.

MATERIALS
1. ¼" felt adhesive.
2. Soft lead marking pencil.
3. Skiving knife.
4. Spray adhesive.

BOUNDARIES
The pad should follow the metatarsal parabola proximally at the metatarsal heads. The medial aspect of the pad follows the first metatarsal shaft posteriorly and superiorly to the talonavicular articulation. The posterior aspect of the pad crosses the foot at the anterior aspect of the calcaneus.

CONSTRUCTION
1. Cut a piece of ¼" adhesive felt into a rectangle 3½" × 7" approximating the size of the foot to be treated.
2. Place the felt pad on the foot so that the back edge rests just anterior to the weight-bearing tuberosity of the calcaneus. The lateral edge of the pad should lie flush with the lateral aspect of the foot.
3. With a soft lead pencil draw a

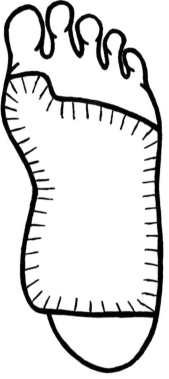

line from just behind the fifth metatarsal head following the metatarsal parabola to a point between the first and second metatarsal heads. Then continue the line distally until the anterior aspect of first metatarsal head is reached. The line then changes direction and continues to the medial plantar edge of the foot. The line then

Berger, O.R.: Orthopedic Padding. *Chiropody Record*, 26 (7): 112-113, 1943.

passes proximally following the medial plantar border of the first metatarsal shaft. At the first metatarsal cuneiform articulation, the line extends superiorly to the talonavicular articulation, then abruptly back inferiorly to the medial plantar edge of the heel. The line continues back across to the lateral edge of the foot and follows the natural contour of the foot distally to the starting point.

4. The pad is cut with sharp scissors along the pencil line.

5. The pad is skived according to the following specifications. The anterior aspect of the pad is skived in the same manner as the Morton's Compensating Pad. The lateral side is skived narrow anteriorly and wider posteriorly. The medial side is skived abruptly along the extension to the first metatarsal cuneiform articulation and much wider to the posterior aspect of the pad. The posterior edge is skived long enough to make the pad fit smoothly and be level with the weight-bearing tuberosity of the calcaneus.

6. Prepare the plantar aspect of the foot with spray adhesive and adhere pad to the foot.

ADDITIONAL COMMENTS
The pad can be easily secured for longer wear by adhering strips of one-inch adhesive tape across the plantar aspect of the foot at various points.

CUBOID PAD

INDICATIONS
To lend support to the outer longitudinal column of the foot, especially in suspected cases of cuboid subluxation.

MATERIALS
⅛" or ¼" adhesive felt and scissors. scissors.

BOUNDARIES
Plantar aspect of cuboid bone.

CONSTRUCTION
1. Cut a rectangle of felt approximately 1½" wide and 2" in length.
2. Trim pad to surface area of plantar aspect of cuboid.
3. If necessary, minimally skive edges.
4. Adhere to plantar aspect of the foot inferior to the cuboid.

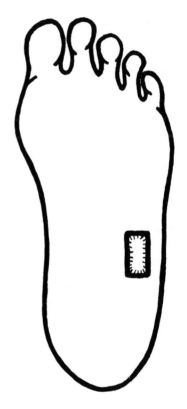

Original contribution by J.C. D'Amico.

THE LONG ARCH PAD

INDICATIONS
Long arch fatigue, symptomatic pes planus, ankle pain, foot strain, plantar fasciitis, any pronatory problems.

MATERIALS
1. ¼" adhesive felt.
2. Soft lead pencil.
3. Skiving knife.
4. Spray adhesive.

BOUNDARIES
The pad follows the fourth intermetatarsal space laterally. The back edge crosses the foot anterior to the weight-bearing tuberosity of the calcaneus, the anterior edge passes proximal to the metatarsal parabola and the medial border passes proximally along the first metatarsal shaft to the first metatarsal cuneiform articulation where it slopes superiorly to the talonavicular articulation. The pad then passes abruptly inferiorly to the medial border of the heel.

CONSTRUCTION
1. Cut a rectangle from ¼" adhesive felt approximately 3½" × 6".
2. Lightly adhere the felt to the foot so that the lateral side of the

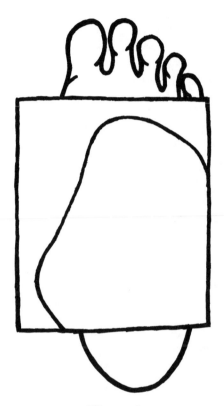

Figure 1.

foot is flush with a 6" edge of felt and the posterior edge rests just proximal to the weight-bearing tuberosity of the calcaneus (Fig. 1).

3. Now with a soft lead pencil mark the shape of the pad by drawing a line just proximal to the metatarsal parabola to a point just between the first and second metatarsal heads. At this point

Berger, O.R.: Orthopedic padding. *Chiropody Record*, 26 (4): 1943, pp. 72, 73, 84.

the line is carried back along the plantar surface of the first metatarsal shaft to the metatarsal cuneiform articulation where it curves superiorly to the talonavicular articulation and then abruptly inferiorly to the medial border of the heel.

4. The pad is now skived with a sharp knife. The lateral side of the pad is skived from about the fourth metatarsal bone and center of the cuboid down to a feather edge with the skive being a bit wider posteriorly. The metatarsal parabola is skived from near the bases of the metatarsal bones forward to a feather edge. The medial side is skived from a point between the bases of the first and second metatarsal bones and the point where the medial flange meets the lateral border of the heel. The back edge of the pad is skived from only ¾" distally and feathered to the back edge (Fig. 2).

5. Prepare the foot with spray adhesive and adhere pad.

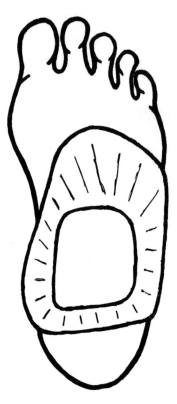

Figure 2.

COMBINATION METATARSAL CUBOID PAD

INDICATIONS
This pad is advantageous in the treatment of Morton's Neuroma.

MATERIALS
1. ¼" felt.
2. Soft lead marking pencil.
3. Skiving knife.

BOUNDARIES
The anterior border follows the metatarsal parabola proximally, the lateral border follows the shaft of the fifth metatarsal proximally where it crosses the foot at the calcaneo cuboid articulation; medially the pad runs anteriorly from the intermediate cuneiform then medially to support the second metatarsal shaft.

CONSTRUCTION
1. Cut the ¼" felt into a shape 2½" wide × 4-5" long.
2. The felt is then placed on the foot so that the lateral edge of the pad rides along the plantar surface of the fifth metatarsal shaft.
3. The anterior aspect of the pad is marked just proximal to the metatarsal heads and the posterior aspect of the pad should extend just behind the calcaneo cuboid articulation.

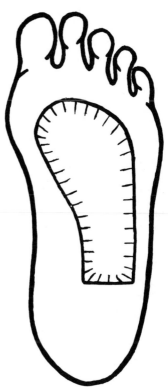

4. The pad should be skived abruptly except on the medial side where skiving is not necessary.
5. In applying the pad to the foot, it should be placed so that the lateral skive falls over the shaft of the fifth metatarsal with the full thickness of the pad giving support to the fourth metatarsal shaft.

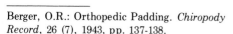

Berger, O.R.: Orthopedic Padding. *Chiropody Record*, 26 (7), 1943, pp. 137-138.

COMBINATION LONG ARCH PAD AND METATARSAL PAD

INDICATIONS
Long arch pain with metatarsal lesions.

MATERIALS
1. ¼" felt, 1" adhesive tape.
2. Soft lead pencil.
3. Skiving knife.

BOUNDARIES
The boundaries for this pad are the same as those indicated for the Long Arch Pad except the skived edges are different.

CONSTRUCTION
1. Cut a piece of ¼" felt approximately 3½" × 6".
2. Place the felt flush against the lateral side of the foot. The back of the pad should rest just in front of the weight bearing tuberosity of the calcaneus.
3. With a marking pencil, scribe a line on the pad starting at the fifth metatarsal head moving medially following the arc of the lesser metatarsal heads. The line is then carried back along the plantar surface of the first metatarsal shaft to the first metatarsal cuneiform articulation. Here it curves superiorly to the talonavicular articulation and then

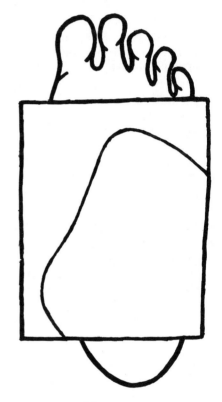

Figure 1.

abruptly inferiorly to the medial border of the heel (Fig. 1).
4. Skive the pad as follows:
   a. Lateral side—From between fourth and fifth metatarsals and center of cuboid outwards to a feather edge.
   b. Anterior side—The length of this abrupt skive is ¼" on ¼" felt.
   c. Medial side—From between first and second metatar-

Berger, O.R.: Orthopedic Padding. *Chiropody Record*, 26 (5), 1943, pp. 87-89.

sal bones and a point where the medial flange meets the medial border of the heel.

d. The posterior skive should be just long enough to be perfectly smooth and level from the unskived part of the pad and on to the weight-bearing tuberosity of the calcaneus (Fig. 2).

5. Place the pad on the foot so that the full thickness of the felt will come directly behind the metatarsal heads and the skived portion will be under the metatarsal heads.

6. This pad can be strapped to the foot with 1″ adhesive tape.

ADDITIONAL COMMENTS

For a flaccid foot, it is necessary to place the pad even further forward to allow for elongation of the foot on weight bearing.

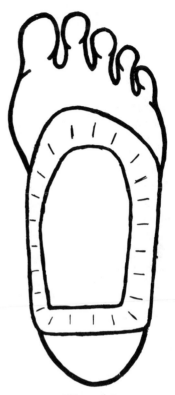

Figure 2.

THE METATARSAL PAD

INDICATIONS
To relieve pressure from painful lesions located at the metatarsal heads.

MATERIALS
1. ¼" adhesive felt.
2. Soft lead pencil.
3. Skiving knife.
4. Adhesive tape or moleskin.

BOUNDARIES
The anterior border follows the metatarsal parabola from a point just proximal to the metatarsal heads. The medial and lateral sides follow the first and fourth interspaces proximally to cross the foot perpendicular to the metatarsals at their bases.

CONSTRUCTION
1. Cut a piece of ¼" felt 3" × 4".
2. Mark the felt pad according to the outline described in the boundary section above.
3. The pad is skived on a 45 degree angle along the medial and lateral sides. The posterior skive should be approximately 1" long and feathered so as to conform with the foot at the tarsal metatarsal junction.
4. Adhere the pad to the foot.

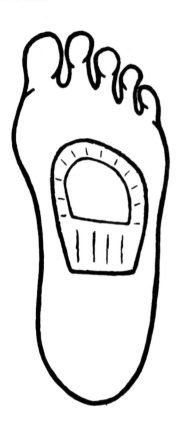

5. Secure with adhesive tape or moleskin.

ADDITIONAL COMMENTS
This pad can be constructed to almost any need.
1. It may be extended forward either full thickness or with a long bevel to cover the three middle metatarsal heads. This variation can include a circular

Berger, O.R.: Orthopedic Padding. *Chiropody Record*, 26 (4), 1943, pp. 89, 90, 101.

aperture to disperse weight away from a particular lesion.

2. The pad can also be constructed as a single or double wing shape isolating the first or fifth metatarsal heads or both with a full width metatarsal pad going completely across the foot.

3. The metatarsal pad can be incorporated into other pads for the plantar surfaces of the foot.

4. The pads can be strapped with adhesive tape encircling the foot just proximal to the metatarsal heads.

REMOVABLE SPENCO METATARSAL PAD

INDICATIONS
The pad can be used to disperse
weight away from any painful plantar lesion.

MATERIALS
1. Spenco.
2. No. 2A tubegauze.
3. Rubber cement.
4. Kidskin leather or vinyl.
5. Dental roll.
6. Liquid latex.
7. 3″ adhesive tape.
8. ¼″ adhesive felt.

BOUNDARIES
The boundaries are to be determined by the podiatrist as any
plantar pad may be constructed using the above materials.

CONSTRUCTION
1. Shape the desired dispersion
   pad from ¼″ adhesive felt with
   an aperture to conform with the
   painful lesion.
2. Prepare the plantar surface of
   the foot with spray adhesive.
3. Lightly adhere the pad in
   place. The adhesive surface of
   the pad is adhered directly to
   the skin (Fig. 1).
4. Using an 8″ length of tubegauze, encircle the dorsal surfaces of toes two, three and four
   and pass the ends of the tubegauze down through the first
   and fourth interspaces. Ad-

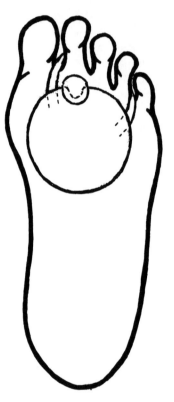

Figure 1.

here the ends of the tubegauze
to the surface of the felt pad
with rubber cement.
   a. For dorsal excrescences on
the toes, a length of dental cotton should be inserted into the
tubegauze before adhering the
ends of the tubegauze to the
felt.
5. The entire outer surface of the
   pad is now covered with 3″ ad-

hesive tape encasing the ends of the tubegauze between the tape and the felt pad (Fig. 2).

6. The entire pad is removed from the foot and the excess adhesive tape is trimmed away.

7. Cut a circular piece of Spenco approximately 1″ larger than the diameter of the aperture in the felt pad.

8. Skive the edges of the Spenco and center the Spenco over the aperture in the felt pad. Adhere the Spenco to the adhesive side of the felt pad.

9. Now apply a coating of rubber cement to both sides of the felt-Spenco appliance.

10. Cover both sides of the appliance with a piece of soft leather or vinyl and trim to shape.

11. Coat the tubegauze section of the appliance with liquid latex and set aside to dry.

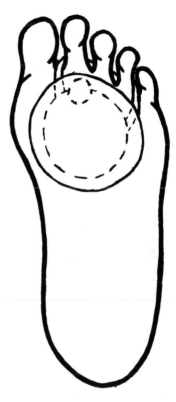

Figure 2.

ADDITIONAL COMMENTS

1. This appliance can be removed and applied to the foot as needed.

2. The life of the appliance can be increased by occasional dusting with talcum powder.

COMBINED FILLER AND METATARSAL PAD WITH VALGUS FLANGE

INDICATIONS
To alleviate discomfort caused by painful lesions on the plantar aspect of the feet.

MATERIALS
1. Inner section of plastizote 6″ × 4″, ⅛″ or ³⁄₁₆″ thickness.
2. Rubazote padding ⅛″ thick in light, standard or heavy density according to requirements.
3. Linen backing or other fabric.
4. Elastic web or alternative type of elastic band.
5. Outer section of plastizote 6″ × 4″, ¹⁄₁₆″ or ⅛″ thickness.
6. Rubber cement.

CONSTRUCTION
Method of construction and sequence of aplication is the same as described for the plastizote hallux valgus shield.
1. Prepare the foot by applying two double thicknesses of 1″ adhesive tape to the plantar surface of the foot, one just proximal to the metatarsal heads, the other just anterior to the weight-bearing tuberosity of the calcaneus (Fig. 1).
2. Felt domes of ⅛″ thickness can be placed over the pressure

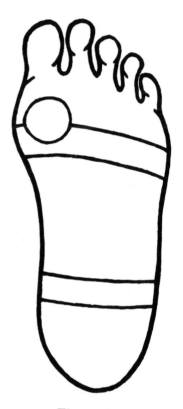

Figure 1.

areas if it is considered necessary to form a deeper cavity.
3. The inner section of plastizote is heated and molded to the plantar surface of the foot making sure one 4″ edge lies just distal to the weight-bearing tuberosity of the calcaneus (Fig. 2).

McDonald, R.: Hand Moulded Plastizote Appliances. *The Chiropodist*, July 1967, pp. 235-239.

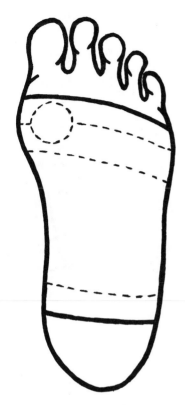

Figure 2.

4. Then coat the inner section with rubber cement.
5. Adhere a double thickness elastoplast strip of desired width (adhesive side to adhesive side) to the inner section. The strip is adhered to the pad on the medial and lateral sides while encircling the dorsum of the foot with moderate tension (Fig. 3).
6. Now fashion the appropriate corex shield for the plantar lesions in question. Coat with rubber cement and adhere to the inner layer of plastizote in the desired position (Fig. 4).
7. Now adhere a 6″ × 4″ linen backing over the entire appliance.
8. Apply rubber cement adhesive over the linen backing.
9. A second piece of plastizote 6″

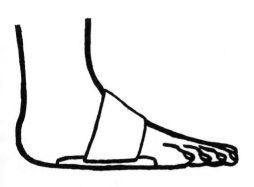

Figure 3.

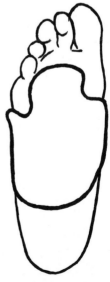

Figure 4.

× 4″ is then heated, prepared with rubber cement, and molded over the structure.

10. The pad is now trimmed with the anterior portion of the pad conforming to the lesions as outlined by the shape of the corex layer (Fig. 5).

11. The pad is now finished by heating the edges as described in the plastizote HAV shield.

ADDITIONAL COMMENTS

The elastoplast band provides easy removal of the pad.

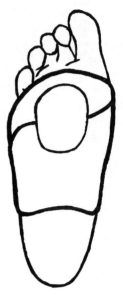

Figure 5.

REMOVABLE DOUBLE WINGED METATARSAL PAD

INDICATIONS
For padding of lesions found under metatarsal heads.

MATERIALS
1. ¼" adhesive foam or felt.
2. No. 1 tubegauze.
3. Moleskin.

BOUNDARIES
The pad is approximately 3" at its widest part. The anterior border runs proximal to the fifth and first metatarsal heads and directly beneath the second, third and fourth metatarsal heads. The posterior portion of the pad crosses the foot at the base of the first metatarsal.

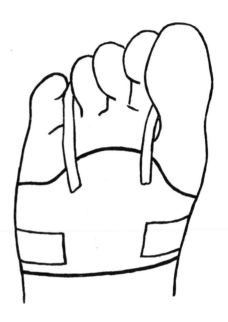

CONSTRUCTION
1. Cut the ¼" foam or felt to the shape as described above.
2. Now cut two strips of No. 1 tubegauze of approximately 6" in length.
3. Place the pad on the plantar surface of the foot with the non-adhesive surface against the skin. Adhere one 6" strip to the adhesive side of the pad. Make sure to adhere both ends to the pad while maintaining tension over the dorsum of the foot. The ends should be adhered at approximately midshaft of the first metatarsal.
4. Adhere the second strip of tubegauze by securing one end to the pad at the fourth interdigital space. Then pass the tubegauze over the dorsum of toes two, three and four, and with slight tension adhere the remaining end to the pad at the first interdigital space.
5. To finish the pad, fashion a piece of moleskin of exact size and shape as the first pad and adhere the moleskin to the pad adhesive side to adhesive side.
6. Trim and skive to desired shape and fit.

Drew, F.A.: Removable Padding. *Current Chiropody*, October 1955, pp. 9-13.

ADDITIONAL COMMENTS

1. This pad can easily be removed and applied whenever necessary.

2. Occasional dusting with talcum powder will increase the life of the pad.

COMBINED METATARSAL PAD WITH TOE LOOP AND HEEL LOOP

INDICATIONS
To protect plantar lesions while exerting a lever action keeping the toes plantarflexed.

MATERIALS
1. ⅛" adhesive foam.
2. ⅛" corex.
3. Chamois leather.
4. Rubber cement.
5. Tubegauze (Nos. 1 or 2A).
6. ¼" rubber dam.

BOUNDARIES
The pad will have the same boundaries as the metatarsal pad while being slung around the three middle toes and the posterior aspect of the heel.

CONSTRUCTION
1. With the adhesive side facing away from the skin, construct a metatarsal pad as described in the instructions given for the basic metatarsal pad using ⅛" adhesive foam. The only variation here is that the anterior aspect of the pad will lie just proximal to the bases of the five toes.
2. Now construct a new metatar-

Charlesworth, Franklin: Combined Metatarsal Pad with Toe Loop and Heel Loop. *British Journal of Chiropody*, 23 (10), 1958, pp. 272-273.

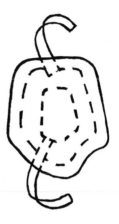

Figure 1.

sal pad of ⅛" corex with proper balancing for the painful areas that is slightly smaller than the foam metatarsal pad.
3. The corex pad is then adhered to the adhesive side of the ⅛" foam pad.
4. Prepare the non-adhesive foam face with rubber cement.
5. Now cut two pieces of chamois leather slightly larger than the foam cushion and cover one side of each chamois with rubber cement.
6. Prepare a toe loop with No. 1 tubegauze to run from the medial distal aspect of the metatarsal pad up through the first interspace around the dorsum of the second, third and

fourth toes, down through the fourth interspace and ending at the lateral distal aspect of the metatarsal pad.

7. Affix the toe loop by sandwiching the ends between the chamois leather and the foam pad (Fig. 1).

8. Prepare the corex pad with rubber cement.

9. Now prepare a heel loop with a length of ¼" rubber dam to run from the medial posterior aspect of the pad around the posterior aspect of the heel and back to the lateral posterior aspect of the pad.

10. Affix the toe loop as described in Step 7 with the second piece of chamois leather.

11. Trim the chamois layers to the dimensions of the adhesive foam.

12. Sling the pad to the foot (Fig. 2).

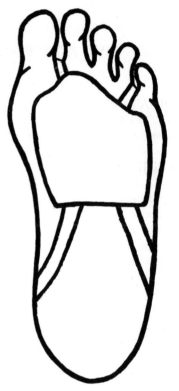

Figure 2.

AN ECONOMICAL METATARSAL PAD

INDICATIONS
For relief of painful plantar lesions.

MATERIALS
1. Discarded pieces of scrap, foam rubber, plastizote, spenco, corex, felt, etc.
2. Linen.
3. No. 1 tubegauze.
4. Moleskin.

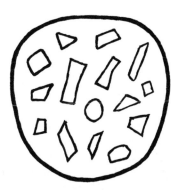

Figure 1.

BOUNDARIES
This pad can be custom made to fit over any lesion that is desired by the podiatrist.

CONSTRUCTION
1. As scrap pieces of padding are collected, adhere the scraps closely together on a linen backing. Try to adhere scrap pieces of equal thickness on the same linen backing.
2. When enough scraps are collected, adhere the entire mass to a piece of moleskin and cut out the desired shape pad to fit your patient's needs (Fig. 1).
3. Construct a No. 1 tubegauze sling that will encircle toes two, three and four and be secured to the pad through the first and fourth interdigital spaces.
4. The ends of the tubegauze and

Simko, Michael V.: Economy in Padding. *Chiropody Record*, 38 (7-8), p. 27.

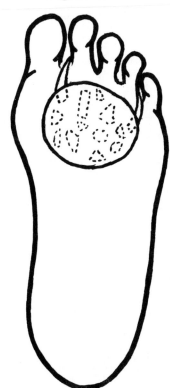

Figure 2.

the scrap pieces are enclosed in
the pad with a second layer of
moleskin. This procedure

should produce an intact pad
that can be slung over the toe
(Fig. 2).

THE PLANTAR COMBINATION PAD

INDICATIONS

A pad to cover a great area of plantar surface while incorporating padding for lesions of individual preference.

MATERIALS

1. ³⁄₁₆″ adhesive felt.
2. 2½″ stockinette.
3. ³⁄₁₆″ or ⁵⁄₁₆″ adhesive foam.
4. ¹⁄₁₆″ adhesive felt or moleskin.

BOUNDARIES

The pad will cover the entire plantar surface of the foot from just proximal to the metatarsal heads to the posterior aspect of the calcaneus.

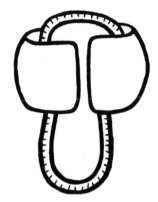

Figure 1.

CONSTRUCTION

1. Using ³⁄₁₆″ adhesive felt construct a pad covering the area on the plantar surface of the foot as instructed by the boundaries above.
2. Skive the adhesive face of the felt on all edges.
3. Cut a metatarsal strap to fit snugly around the dorsum of the forefoot. This is accomplished by adhering a piece of 2½″ wide stockinette to the adhesive face of the pad while the non-adhesive face of the pad is posi-

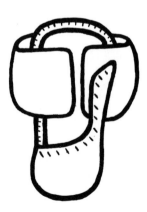

Figure 2.

Dowdeswell-Childs, T.G.: Replaceable Padding for Geriatrics, Part I. *The Chiropodist*, 21 1), January 1966, pp. 4-7.

tioned on the plantar surface of the foot (Fig. 1).

4. Now fashion a custom pad for the lesions to be treated from ³⁄₁₆″ or ⁵⁄₁₆″ adhesive foam.

5. Adhere the finished pad in position on the original pad adhesive face to adhesive face (Fig. 2).

6. With a piece of ¹⁄₁₆″ adhesive felt or moleskin, cut a shape that will fill the remaining area left by the application of the custom pad.

7. Trim and skive all remaining edges (Fig. 3).

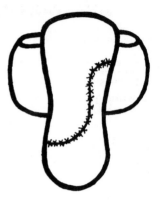

Figure 3.

METATARSAL BAND WITH PLANTAR PAD

INDICATIONS
To decrease the width of a splay foot while padding plantar metatarsal lesions.

MATERIALS
1. ¼" adhesive felt or adhesive foam.
2. 3" elastoplast.
3. No. 1 tubegauze.

BOUNDARIES
The elastoplast encircles the five metatarsal shafts completely. The elastoplast strip is slung to the foot over the second, third and fourth toes.

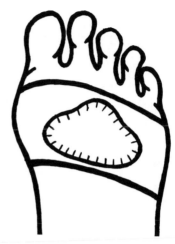

Figure 1.

CONSTRUCTION
1. A strapping of 3" elastoplast is made to encircle the foot with tension at the metatarsal shafts. The strap is adhered to itself on the dorsum of the foot. The adhesive face of the elastoplast is away from the skin.
2. A custom metatarsal pad, no more than 3" from its most distal aspect to its most proximal aspect, is fashioned from ¼" adhesive foam or felt.
3. The custom pad is then adhered in place on to the adhesive side of the elastoplast strap at the plantar surface of the foot (Fig. 1).

Dowdeswell-Childs, T.G.: Replaceable Padding for Geriatrics, Part I. *The Chiropodist*, 21 (1), January 1966, pp. 6-7.

4. A piece of No. 1 tubegauze is cut with sufficient length to wrap about the dorsum of toes two, three and four and pass plantarly through toe spaces one and four.
5. With moderate tension the tubegauze is adhered to the elastoplast strap on the plantar surface of the foot.
6. Now a second strap of 3" elastoplast is laid over the first strap adhesive face to adhesive face. This strap will serve to sandwich the ends of the tubegauze sling and the metatarsal pad snugly to the other elastoplast strap. The ends of this strap will also overlap and adhere dorsally (Fig. 2).

ADDITIONAL COMMENTS

1. The use of an arrow marker at a designated toe will enable the patient to fit the pad properly for future wearings.
2. Occasional dusting with talcum powder will increase the life of the pad.

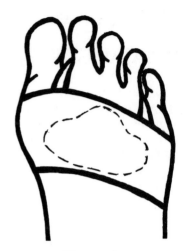

Figure 2.

METATARSAL SHAFTS FOR INTERDIGITAL CORNS

INDICATIONS

For relief of pressure between two toes which are causing helome molle or for individual metatarsal head lesions.

MATERIALS

1. ⅛", ³⁄₁₆" or ¼" felt.
2. Adhesive tape.
3. Skiving knife.
4. Moleskin.

BOUNDARIES

The felt shaft will form a crescent just proximal to the lesion and extend posteriorly directly beneath the metatarsal shaft to the metatarsal base.

CONSTRUCTION

1. Cut a piece of adhesive felt (thickness may vary according to amount of depth necessary) approximately ¾" wide and 3½" long.
2. Cut a crescentic aperture in one end of the felt shaft that will accommodate the painful lesion (Fig. 1).
3. Skive all edges except the end of the felt that contains the aperture.
4. This pad is now secured to the foot by application of a piece of moleskin that approximates the shape of the traditional metatarsal pad. Make sure the pad lies directly beneath the meta-

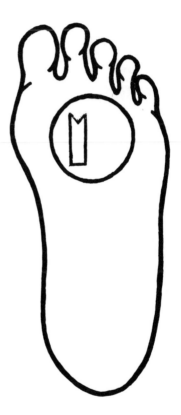

Figure 1.

tarsal bone with the crescentic aperture hugging the lession (Fig. 2).

ADDITIONAL COMMENTS

These shafts can be transferred for use at the intermetatarsal spaces to relieve pain due to intermetatarsal neuroma by spreading the respective metatarsals apart on weight bearing.

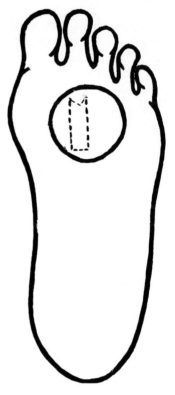

Figure 2.

PARALLEL STRIP PADDING

INDICATIONS
To distribute weight and pressure away from painful lesions on the plantar surface of the foot.

MATERIALS
1. According to individual preference, adhesive felt of varying thickness can be used.
2. Moleskin.

BOUNDARIES
The pads are placed in parallel formation. The length and width of the pad is determined by the area to be protected.

CONSTRUCTION
1. Locate the lesion to be protected and by palpation determine the thickness of the pad to be used.
2. Now cut two strips of adhesive felt of exactly the same rectangular shape and size. The finished rectangle should be long enough to extend at least ½" distal and proximal to the lesion. The width of the strip should be at least ½".
3. Align the two pads in parallel position by adhering them to the foot. The pads should buttress

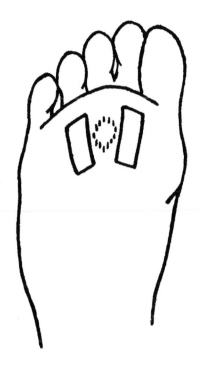

the lesion on both sides and lie with the long axis of the pad facing in an anterior-posterior direction.
4. Cover both parallel strips with a piece of moleskin that approximates the shape and size of a metatarsal pad.

Sansone, Ralph E.: Parallel Strip Padding for Weight Stress Distribution and Redirection. *J.A.P.A.*, 60 (5), May 1970, pp. 193-198.

A SUSTAINED FULL LENGTH PLANTAR PAD

INDICATIONS

To construct a pad that will fit easily into the shoe with a longer life than ordinary padding.

MATERIALS

1. Adhesive foam.
2. Adhesive felt.
3. ⅛" corex or leather.
4. Rubber cement.
5. Skiving knife.
6. Moleskin.

BOUNDARIES

The pad fits into the shoe and will be the same shape as the entire plantar surface of the foot.

CONSTRUCTION

1. Cut a rectangular "blank" of ⅛" corex or leather that approximates the size and shape of the plantar surface of the foot. The pad should extend from the toe sulcus to the posterior aspect of the heel.
2. The "blank" is now placed in the shoe for one week so that the foot and associated excrescences will leave an impression.
3. The "blank" can now be trimmed and cut to desired shape. For additional comfort, adhesive felt or foam of varying thickness may be added to the "blank" where desired. The finished blank can also be hollowed in desired areas or even be perforated to accommodate for painful lesions.

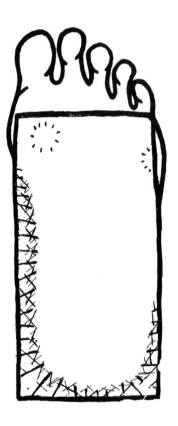

4. The pad is finished by sandwiching the entire appliance in moleskin.
5. Trim to fit and place in the shoe.

REPLACEABLE PLANTAR COVER

INDICATIONS
For plantar lesions causing pain which require a removable appliance.

MATERIALS
1. No. 6 roll foam.
2. ¹⁄₁₆″ adhesive felt.
3. No. 1 tubegauze.
4. Moleskin.
5. Corex, ¼″ or ⅛″ adhesive felt or foam.

BOUNDARIES
The appliance encircles the hallux and covers the plantar surface of the foot from the toe sulcus to the base of the metatarsals.

CONSTRUCTION
1. With sharp scissors, slit the edge of an 8″ length of No. 6 roll foam leaving intact a portion that can slide over and encircle the entire hallux (Fig. 1).
2. Cut a piece of ¹⁄₁₆″ adhesive felt that will be slightly larger than the entire cut portion of the roll foam when unrolled to a flat sheet.
3. Cut a length of No. 1 tubegauze which can sling over the fourth toe. The ends are then firmly pressed in place on the adhesive

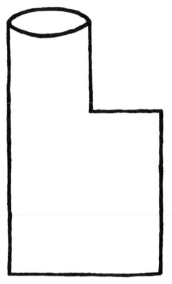

Figure 1.

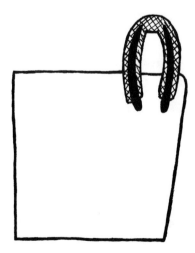

Figure 2.

Dowdeswell-Childs, T.G.: Replaceable Padding for Geriatrics, Part II. *The Chiropodist*, 21 (1), February 1966, p 34.

side of the $\frac{1}{16}''$ felt. To avoid stretching the tubegauze, a length of $\frac{1}{2}''$ adhesive tape can be applied to the tubegauze loop (Fig. 2).

4. Now a pad can be fashioned from corex, adhesive foam, adhesive felt, etc. to accommodate for any plantar lesion. The pad is then adhered in place to the roll foam (Fig. 3).

5. The roll foam is now pressed onto the adhesive face of the $\frac{1}{16}''$ felt with the loop in position to sling over the fourth toe.

6. The exposed plantar surface of roll foam may now be covered with a layer of moleskin creating a sandwich effect for the entire roll foam appliance.

7. Trim all rough edges and apply to foot slinging the roll foam over the hallux and the tubegauze over the fourth toe (Fig. 4).

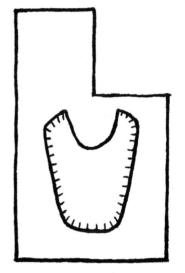

Figure 3.

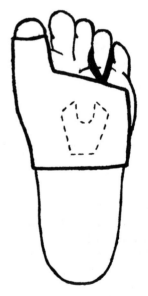

Figure 4.

PERMANENT SPONGE RUBBER SNAP-ON PAD

INDICATIONS
To construct a resilient, hygienic, non-allergic, removable plantar pad.

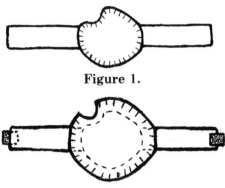

Figure 1.

MATERIALS
1. ¼ " adhesive foam.
2. ⅙" rubber dam.
3. Velcro.
4. Moleskin.
5. Rubber cement.

Figure 2.

BOUNDARIES
The strapping will encircle the foot at the metatarsal shafts to anchor the pad. The pad itself approximates the shape of a conventional metatarsal pad.

CONSTRUCTION
1. Using ¼ " adhesive foam, fashion an oval which is approximately 3″ long and 2″ wide. The oval is skived and apertures may be cut into the edge of the pad to accommodate for plantar metatarsal head lesions.
2. Cut two strips of ¹⁄₁₆″ rubber dam 3½″ long by 1″ wide.
3. Adhere the rubber dam strips to the edges of the adhesive foam at the long axis. This should produce an appliance which looks similar to a wrist watch (Fig. 1).

4. Now adhere with rubber cement a piece of velcro to the remaining free ends of the rubber dam. A velcro piece is adhered to the underside of one rubber dam strip. The other velcro piece is adhered to the remaining rubber dam so that the two velcro strips will face each other for fastening purposes.
5. Using moleskin construct two ovals slightly larger in size than the adhesive foam oval. Incorporate the adhesive foam pad between the two moleskin ovals.
6. Trim all edges with scissors (Fig. 2).
7. The pad can now be fitted over the forefoot and secured with the velcro fasteners.

ADDITIONAL COMMENTS
The pad is adjustable and will fit on to any size foot.

Rosenstein, Henry: Construction of a Permanent and Hygienic Metatarsal Pad. *The Chiropodist*, 3 (2), February 1948, pp. 32-34.

TRIGGER PADS FOR PLANTAR FOOT SYMPTOMATOLOGY

INDICATIONS

These pads may be used for plantar excrescences, rheumatoid arthritis, neurovascular excrescences, sprains, osteoarthritis, trauma and muscle cramping.

MATERIALS

1. ¼″, ³⁄₁₆″, ⅛″ adhesive latex foam.
2. Adhesive tape.

BOUNDARIES

The locations of these Trigger Pads are determined by palpation on the plantar surface of the foot.

Trigger Point No. 1: Medial side of the second metatarsal head at the condyle pressing in a lateral superior direction.

Trigger Point No. 2: The lateral side of the fourth metatarsal head pressing medially and superiorly.

Trigger Point No. 3: Medial side of the third metatarsal head.

Other less commonly used trigger points are as follows: Behind the second metatarsal head, the second metatarsal phalangeal joint, and second proximal phalanx, behind the fourth metatarsal head, the fourth metatarsal phalangeal joint, shaft of the fourth proximal phalanx, first metatarsal phalangeal joint and fifth metatarsal phalangeal joint.

In the long arch trigger points are

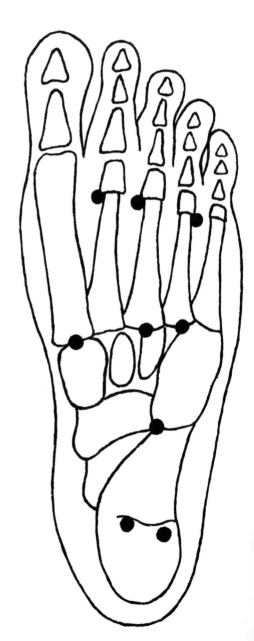

located at the tarsal articulations and the medial, central and lateral aspects of the anterior part of the weight-bearing portion of the heel. Trigger points are also located in the heel itself and occasionally on the dorsum of the foot.

CONSTRUCTION

1. Palpate the trigger points as described above by pressing in lateral, medial or superior direction. If pain is elicited, you have detected a trigger point.
2. Upon finding a trigger point, mark the point on a reference card; + for very sensitive, − for less sensitive.
3. Using a foam rubber dome-shaped pad, adhere the pad on the foot and secure with adhesive tape. The pads are placed on various points proximal or distal to the trigger points palpated.
4. a. For a pad that is placed behind the second or third metatarsal heads, an oblong pad is used with the flange pointing proximally. The pad is cut from a $3/8''$ × $1/2''$ × $1''$ foam rubber wedge.
   b. For pads placed on the second or third proximal phalanges, use oval shaped foam padding. Cut the foam from a $1/4''$ × $3/8''$ × $5/8''$ foam wedge.
   c. Use a crescent shape for padding the proximal phalanx of the hallux.
   d. For mid-plantar and heel symptoms, use an oval shaped heel pad placed on the weight-bearing surface of the calcaneus. This pad can be cut from a $3/16''$ × $7/8''$ × $1 3/8''$ wedge.
   e. Infrequently, when palpation reveals non-sensitive results, a small pad of $3/16''$ thick foam rubber is placed under the cuboid.

ADDITIONAL COMMENTS

1. All pads are placed on non-sensitive areas only. This can be tested by pressing them firmly on the foot before adhering to the foot. If pain is elicited, the pad cannot be used there.
2. As the patient returns (once weekly or twice weekly for sensitive areas), the pads are pressed firmly to check for comfort. If comfort is not achieved, another trigger point is selected.
3. Treatments continue until trigger points are rendered less sensitive and related symptoms subside.
4. After the patient is rendered asymptomatic, the pads are affixed on $1/8''$ foam on a cloth backing cut in the shape of an insole, covered with moleskin and then adhered to the shoe with rubber cement.
5. In less sensitive cases, the pads may be incorporated into leather appliances covered with soft kid leather.
6. This type of padding technique is contraindicated in certain neurological disorders, PVD and arthritic cases where

nerve irritability or degeneration is great.

7. These pads can only be used in shoes that fit adequately and not in high heel shoes because they defeat the purpose of trigger padding in highly sensitive forefoot or midtarsal areas due to abnormal pressure.

8. Women should use medium heel height, low shank shoes for best results.

9. These pads are not to be used with other standard appliances.

10. If a patient is already wearing an appliance, a well skived oblong piece of 3/16″ felt placed on the foot behind the metatarsal heads and extending to the weight-bearing surface of the heel, incorporating the trigger pads, can be used until only the pads alone can be tolerated.

Krout, Robert R.: A Common Source of Foot Symptomatology. *Current Podiatry*, 10 (9), Sept. 1961, pp. 9-14.

_____. A Common Source of Foot Symptomatology. *Current Podiatry*, 10 (10), Oct. 1961, pp. 17-19.

_____. A Common Source of Foot Symptomatology. *Current Podiatry*, 10 (11), Nov. 1961, pp. 18-23.

_____. Shock Absorbing Pads for Symptomatic Feet. *Current Podiatary*, Dec. 1975, pp. 8-12.

THE DANCER'S PAD

INDICATIONS
Symptomatic plantarflexed first ray, first metatarsal bursitis, tibial or fibular sesamoiditis.

MATERIALS
¼" adhesive felt or adhesive foam, scissors, spray adhesive.

BOUNDARIES
The pad assumes the same shape and size of the metatarsal pad. However, the Dancer's Pad has an aperture at the medial, distal edge that begins distally between the first and second metatarsal heads and curves medially to meet the medial side of the pad approximately 1½ cm. proximal to the first metatarsal head.

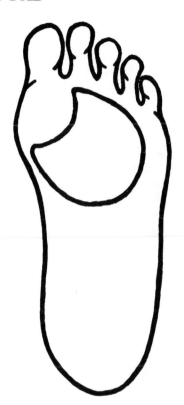

CONSTRUCTION
1. Construct a simple metatarsal pad from ¼" adhesive foam or adhesive felt.
2. Cut an aperture in the pad to allow for weight distribution away from the first metatarsal head as described in the BOUNDARIES section above.
3. Prepare the plantar surface of the foot with spray adhesive.
4. Adhere the pad in place with the distal end of the pad lying just proximal to the metatarsal head.

ADDITIONAL COMMENTS
1. The pad can be affixed to the plantar surface of the foot by binding it down with either moleskin, adhesive tape or paper tape as indicated.
2. The aperture for this pad can also be placed on the lateral aspect of the pad to disperse weight away from the head of the fifth metatarsal as in the case of a painful tailor's bunion, hyperkeratotic lesion, etc.

THE MAYO PAD

INDICATIONS
This pad is used in cases of symptomatic cavus type feet where support under the long arch is necessary.

MATERIALS
1. ¼" adhesive felt.
2. Adhesive tape.
3. Soft lead pencil.
4. Skiving knife.

BOUNDARIES
It is an oblong pad which extends from the medial inferior border of the weight-bearing area of the heel to just behind the first metatarsal head.

CONSTRUCTION
1. Cut a piece of ¼" felt into a 3½" × 5" rectangle. (When more correction is necessary, a double thickness of ¼" felt may be used.)
2. Now lightly adhere the pad to the foot so that the lateral edge of the pad falls over the fourth interspace and the posterior edge of the pad is just proximal to the weight-bearing tuberosity of the calcaneus.
3. Now with a soft lead pencil, mark the shape of the pad by drawing a line just proximal to

the metatarsal parabola to a point just between the first and second metatarsal heads. The line is now carried proximal and superior to the first metatarsal cuneiform articulation then sloping inferiorly again back to the medial border of the heel.
4. The pad is skived leaving an equal slope on all sides with a full-thickness oblong area in the center of the pad.

Berger, O.R.: Orthopedic Padding. *Chiropody Record*, 26 (7), 1943, p. 139.

5. In placing the pad on the foot, one half of the full-thickness area should go on the plantar surface and one half should extend up the medial side of the foot.

ADDITIONAL COMMENTS

The pad can be secured to the foot for longer wear by adhering 1″ strips of adhesive tape at various points along the length of the pad.

V

HALLUX

SIMPLE NONREMOVABLE BUNION SHIELD

INDICATIONS
For painful excrescence or bursitis on the medial or dorsal aspect of the first metatarsal phalangeal joint.

MATERIALS
1. ¼" or ⅛" adhesive foam or adhesive felt.
2. Moleskin.

BOUNDARIES
The pad will encircle one half the proximal aspect of the excrescence and extend proximally on the medial aspect of the foot approximately 1 to 1½ inches.

CONSTRUCTION
1. Scissor cut a piece of adhesive foam or felt into a rectangle 1" × 1½" (the depth of the material should be at the same level as the excrescence when placed on the skin).
2. Cut a semicircular crescent into the felt at one end that approximates the outer border of the excrescence.
3. Taper the opposite end of the

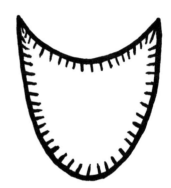

Figure 1.

felt with scissors so it assumes the shape of half an oval.
4. Skive the entire pad leaving the greatest depth at the area of the crescent (Fig. 1).
5. Adhere the pad to the skin with the oval end facing proximally on the medial aspect of the first metatarsal.
6. Fashion a piece of moleskin approximating the shape of the pad allowing ¼" overlap on all borders and adhere directly to the pad.

ADDITIONAL COMMENTS
The pad can be fashioned to accommodate any lesion on the medial or lateral side of the foot.

Schuster, Otto: Foot Orthopaedics. *First Institute of Podiatry*, 1927, pp. 286-288.

PARALLEL STRIP PADDING

INDICATIONS
The pads are used to protect inflamed tissue at any area of the first metatarsal phalangeal joint by diverting presssure away from the areas of irritation.

MATERIALS
¼″, ⅛″ or ³⁄₁₆″ adhesive felt (according to depth of lesion).

BOUNDARIES
These pads will act as buttresses which will lie parallel to the lesion in question on its proximal and distal aspects.

CONSTRUCTION
1. Cut two rectangles of chosen thickness from the adhesive felt. The rectangles should be approximately 1″ × 1½″.

Sansone, Ralph E.: Parallel Strip Padding for Weight Stress Distribution and Redirection. *J.A.P.A.*, 60 (5), May 1970, pp. 193-198.

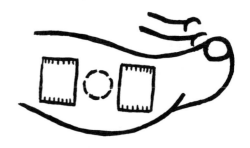

Figure 1.

2. Skive both pads at the 1″ ends.
3. Now place one pad just proximal to the bunion. The long side of the pad will lie next to the lesion perpendicular to the long axis of the first ray.
4. The second pad is placed at the distal aspect of the bunion and parallel to the proximal pad (Fig. 1).

AN INGENIOUS PAD
(FOR BUNIONS OR METATARSALS)

INDICATONS

This pad will alleviate discomfort due to painful plantar lesions about the metatarsal heads or can be utilized as a bunion pad.

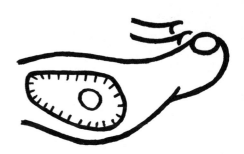

MATERIALS

1. Dependent upon the degree of correction, either ⅛″, ¼″ or ½″ adhesive felt.
2. Skin marking solution.
3. Scissors.

BOUNDARIES

The pad is fabricated as a metatarsal pad approximating the metatarsal parabola distally, and extending to the base of the metatarsals proximally, the medial and lateral borders will approximate the level of the first and fourth interspaces respectively.

CONSTRUCTION

1. Construct a metatarsal pad using the borders as explained above.
2. Stain the lesion created by the bunion with the appropriate solution.

3. The metatarsal pad is now placed against the bunion adhesive side away from the skin to enable transfer of the position of the lesion on to the pad.
4. Now pierce the pad with scissors at the lesion marking and cut a circular aperture out of the felt approximating the size of the lesion.
5. The pad is now adhered over the lesion so that the long axis of the pad is parallel to the long axis of the first ray.
6. The adhered pad should encircle the first ray on medial, dorsal and plantar sides to afford maximum protection from outside pressure.

ADDITIONAL COMMENTS

This pad may also be used as a basic metatarsal pad.

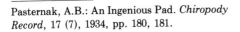

Pasternak, A.B.: An Ingenious Pad. *Chiropody Record*, 17 (7), 1934, pp. 180, 181.

REMOVABLE FELT BUNION SHIELD

INDICATIONS

To relieve pressure on the in-flamed hallux joint and fill the empty space around the ex-crescence.

Figure 1.

MATERIALS

1. ⅛" or ¼" non-adhesive felt (depending upon the depth of the lesion).
2. ⅛" adhesive felt.
3. Moleskin.
4. Sharp scissors.
5. Indelible marking pen.

Figure 2.

BOUNDARIES

The medial aspect of the first MPJ from a point ½" proximal to the joint. The pad will encircle the base of the great toe as well.

CONSTRUCTION

1. Cut a rectangle 2½" × 3½" from the non-adhesive felt. Thickness will depend upon the height of the lesion (Fig. 1).
2. Now fold the rectangle perpendicular to the long axis, with the fold lying one inch from the short side.
3. With sharp scissors cut a half circle at the fold. The diameter of the semicircle should be slightly larger than the diameter of the lesion (Fig. 2).
4. Now unfold the felt rectangle and place the aperture of the pad over the lesion leaving the long unfinished portion of the rectangle to face distally on the medial aspect of the foot.
5. With an indelible marking pen place a reference mark on the felt at the area where the great toe meets the foot.
6. With sharp scissors cut a crescent at the reference mark. The crescent should be approximately ¼" wide at its widest point. The concave border of the crescent should be parallel to the circumference of the circular aperture that surrounds the lesion (Fig. 3).

Polokoff, Morton: Felt Pads for the Bunion Joints 1st and 5th. *Current Chiropody*, February 1954, pp. 11, 12.

7. Sling the pad around the base of the hallux by opening the crescent to accommodate the great toe.

8. The pad is now removed from the foot and is trimmed and skived where necessary to insure proper fit. The entire pad should approximate the shape of an oval when trimming is completed.

9. The distal portion of the bunion aperture is now built up with properly sized $\frac{1}{8}''$ adhesive felt. The adhesive felt is affixed to the pad to approximate the height of the lesion.

10. Skive all edges of the affixed felt until a smooth taper is obtained.

11. The entire pad is now sandwiched between two pieces of moleskin and cut to proper size. Be sure to cut the moleskin leaving an aperture for the excrescence (Fig. 4).

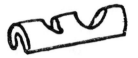

Figure 3.

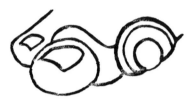

Figure 4.

ADDITIONAL COMMENTS

On subsequent visits the appliance may be made more durable by coating it with silicone.

REMOVABLE FLASK-SHAPED BUNION PAD

INDICATIONS
To alleviate discomfort at the first metatarsal head for prolonged periods of time.

MATERIALS
1. No. 1 tube gauze.
2. ⅛″ felt.
3. ¹⁄₁₆″ felt.
4. Scissors.
5. Skiving knife.

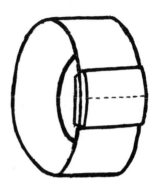

Figure 1.

BOUNDARIES
The pad will extend from the medial aspect of the first metatarsal phalangeal articulation distally and will be secured at the base of the hallux.

CONSTRUCTION
Construction consists of two parts which join together; the first section is in the form of a collar which passes around the large toe.

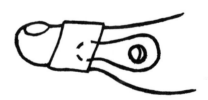

Figure 2.

1. Cut a length of No. 1 tube gauze approximately ¼″ smaller than the circumference of the proximal aspect of the hallux.
2. Then, using a one-inch square of ¹⁄₁₆″ adhesive felt, adhere the tube gauze end to end across the felt forming a loop with the tube gauze (Fig. 1).
3. Now using a second one-inch

square of ¹⁄₁₆″ adhesive felt, adhere the loop (adhesive side to adhesive side) to the other felt square. This should leave a loop of tube gauze enclosed in two adhesive felt squares.
4. The collar is then fitted over the hallux leaving the felt "sandwich" to lie in the first interspace.
5. The second section is fabricated by fashioning a flask-shaped

Davis, A.: A Removable Bunion Pad. *The Chiropody Review*, 12 (3), March 1951, pp. 57-60.

oval pad approximately 2½"
long from the ⅛" adhesive felt.
When the shape is cut make sure
there is sufficient felt both
proximal and distal to the lesion to provide adequate protection.
6. The narrow neck of the flask-
shaped felt is then slipped under the tube gauze loop, adhesive side facing away from the
skin, and adhered to the underside of the loop. Leave one-half
of the width of the tube gauze
free (Fig. 2).
7. The entire pad is now removed
from the foot. A second flask-
shaped loop (the same size as
the first) is cut and adhered (adhesive to adhesive) over the
other flask-shaped pad.
8. Using sharp scissors cut an
aperture through the flask-
shaped pad, at the wide end, to

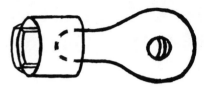

Figure 3.

approximate the size of the lesion.
9. The pad is then trimmed and
skived to individual liking and
secured over the hallux (Fig. 3).

ADDITIONAL COMMENTS
Further adjustments in thickness
at vital points can be made by adhering crescents of felt at the proximal and distal areas of the aperture before adhering the outer felt
flask-shape to the one in direct contact with the foot.

REMOVABLE BUNION PAD WITH FIGURE EIGHT LOOP

INDICATIONS
To protect the bunion from external pressure.

MATERIALS
1. 1" elastoplast.
2. 1" adhesive tape.
3. Non-adhesive felt.
4. Scissors.

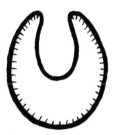

Figure 1.

BOUNDARIES
The pad will encircle the excrescence proximally and the binding wraps about the entire proximal phalanx of the hallux.

CONSTRUCTION
1. Cut a piece of felt of desired thickness into a crescentic shape. The concave border of the crescent is to lie about the proximal aspect of the bunion (as described on page 68) (Fig. 1).
2. Cut a strip of ½" elastoplast 6" long and a piece of adhesive tape of same length.
3. Affix one end of the elastoplast strip to the plantar edge of the crescent with adhesive side away from the skin (Fig. 2).
4. Now hold the pad in place against the medial side of the foot at the proximal aspect of the bunion excrescence while

Figure 2.

winding the strip over the dorsum of the hallux down through the first interspace and back up on the medial side of the hallux. The other end of the strip is affixed to the dorsal tip of the crescent, adhesive side facing away from the skin. The entire pro-

Endersby, M.E.: Removable Hallux Valgus Pad. *The Chiropodist*, 4 (3), 1949, pp. 66-67.

cedure is performed using moderate tension. The result should produce a figure eight loop with the pad adhered to it.

5. Now affix the 1″ adhesive strip directly over the elastoplast strip and follow figure eight loop around, adhering the adhesive faces to each other. This should result in a sandwiching of the felt crescent's tips between the elastoplast and adhesive tape strips.

6. The figure eight loop can be secured to the foot by sliding the loop over the hallux into the first interspace (Fig. 3).

ADDITIONAL COMMENTS

If you wish the pad to be non-re-

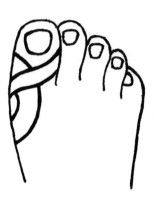

Figure 3.

movable, a simple 1″ binder of elastoplast encircling the foot and pad at the level of the metatarsal heads will suffice.

HALLUX PAD WITH INTERDIGITAL WEDGE

INDICATIONS
To shield the prominence of the first MPJ against shoe pressure while separating the hallux from the second toe.

MATERIALS
1. ¼" adhesive felt or sponge rubber.
2. 3" adhesive tape.
3. Moleskin or elastoplast.

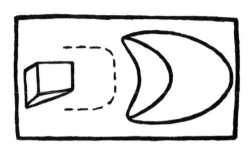

Figure 1.

BOUNDARIES
The medial proximal aspect of the first MPJ and first interspace.

CONSTRUCTION
(Two different pads are to be constructed and incorporated into one appliance.)
1. The first pad is constructed of ¼" felt and made to fit as a tapered crescent about the proximal aspect of the excrescence at the first MPJ (refer to page 68).
2. A second pad is fabricated of ¼" felt as a small wedge. The felt is first cut to ¼" × ½" × ⅜" dimensions.
3. The cube is then tapered along one ⅜" edge creating a wedge that will later be placed in the first interdigital space.

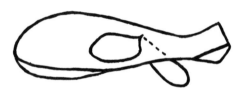

Figure 2.

4. The two pads are then placed on the adhesive side of a 4" strip of tape. The pads are placed 1½" apart with the concave end of pad one facing the tapered edge of pad two (Fig. 1).
5. Now a second piece of tape, the same size as the first, is placed face down (adhesive side to adhesive side) on the first piece of adhesive tape. This procedure will sandwich the two pads within the two pieces of tape.
6. Press the tapes together covering all sides of the two pads and

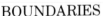

Koppe, W.P.: Palliative Padding and Strapping. *Clin Journal of Chiropody, Podiatry and Pedic Surgery*, 6 (1), 1933, pp. 7-8.

trim all taped edges leaving the two pads connected by a strip between the concave face of the first pad and the tapered edge of the second pad.

7. Cut the strip creating a "U"-shaped opening in the tape. The "U" should face towards and approximate the size and shape of the convex crescent in the bunion pad and be just large enough to accept the first toe.

8. This will form a flap which is then turned backwards towards the wedge leaving an aperture for the first toe (Fig. 2).

9. The pad is then worn with the wedge in the first interspace and the crescent pad lies proximal to the bunion deformity (Fig. 3).

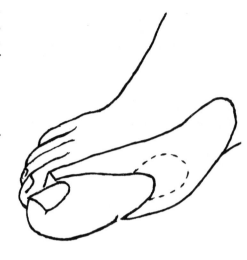

Figure 3.

ADDITIONAL COMMENTS

Moleskin or elastoplast may be used in lieu of adhesive tape.

REPLACEABLE ROLL FOAM HAV SHIELD

INDICATIONS

To transfer weight and pressure away from a painful bunion.

MATERIALS

1. No. 6 rollfoam.
2. $^{3}/_{16}$" adhesive foam rubber.
3. Spray adhesive.
4. No. 2A tubegauze.

BOUNDARIES

The pad will encircle the entire hallux and extend proximally to cover the medial aspect of the foot to the middle of the first metatarsal.

CONSTRUCTION

1. Cut a length of No. 6 rollfoam sufficiently long enough to cover the large toe and extend 1½" proximal to the first MPJ.
2. Split the foam tube along one side so that enough intact foam tubing remains to completely cover the entire large toe.
3. Now an aperture can be cut in the rollfoam sufficiently large enough to accommodate the bunion (Fig. 1).
4. Fashion a $^{3}/_{16}$" adhesive foam crescent to border the proximal aspect of the aperture in the rollfoam and adhere in place over the exterior of the pad.

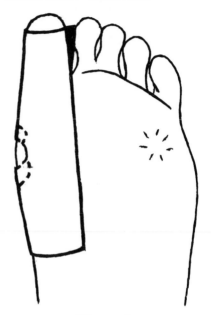

Figure 1.

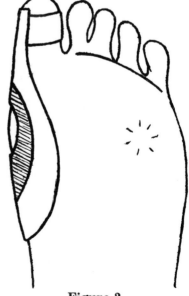

Figure 2.

Dowdeswell-Childs, T.G.: Replaceable Padding for Geriatrics, Part II. *The Chiropodist*, 21 (1), February 1966, pp. 36, 37.

5. Spray the entire exterior of the pad with adhesive spray.
6. The entire pad is now covered with No. 2A tubegauze, which is cut in the same manner as the rollfoam; this procedure will en-case the adhesive foam crescent within the rollfoam and stockinette.
7. Trim to fit and slip the entire pad over the hallux (Fig. 2).

LONG LASTING REMOVABLE HAV SHIELD

INDICATIONS
To protect a painful bunion deformity from excessive pressure.

MATERIALS
1. ³⁄₁₆″ adhesive foam rubber.
2. Moleskin.
3. No. 2A tubegauze.

BOUNDARIES
The pad will sling over the large toe and cover an area approximately ¾″ distal to the first MPJ and 1½″ proximal to the first MPJ.

CONSTRUCTION
1. Using sharp scissors, cut a piece of ³⁄₁₆″ foam rubber into the shape of an oval. The oval should be at least 3″ long and 1¾″ wide.
2. Now cut a concave crescent into the widest area of the oval pad to accommodate the bunion excrescence.
3. Using scissors cut a piece of moleskin of the same shape as the adhesive foam oval. The moleskin piece should overlap the adhesive foam approximately ¼″ on all borders.
4. While holding the nonadhesive side of the moleskin against the medial side of the foot, affix the non-adhesive face of the foam pad to the moleskin. The crescent should fit proximal to the bunion. Allow ¼″ overlap on all sides.

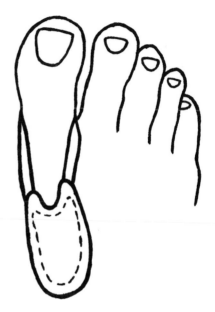

Figure 1.

5. Using a 1½-2″ length of tubegauze, adhere one end to the dorsal tip of the crescent and pass the tubegauze down through the first interspace slinging the hallux while adhering the remaining end of the tubegauze to the plantar tip of the crescent.
6. Fashion a second piece of moleskin of exact size and shape as the first piece and adhere directly over the pad on the foot. This should produce a finished pad with adhesive foam and tubegauze encased within.
7. Trim all edges to desired fit (Fig. 1).

REMOVABLE LATEX HAV PAD

INDICATIONS
To alleviate pain due to dorsal or medial heloma durum found at the first MPJ.

MATERIALS
1. ¼" adhesive foam.
2. ¹⁄₁₆" latex sheeting.

BOUNDARIES
To surround a dorsal or medial excrescence at the first MPJ while slung to the great toe.

CONSTRUCTION
1. Cut two rectangles of 3" × 2" dimensions from the ¼" adhesive foam.
2. Place the foam pieces together non-adhesive side to non-adhesive side and round off all corners to approximate an oval shape. Make sure to retain the length and width of the foam rectangles.
3. Lightly adhere only the tapered ends of the oval.
4. Now wrap a length of ¹⁄₁₆" latex sheeting, that is approximately ¼" wide, through the first interspace and around the hallux.
5. The free ends can be inserted into the wide end of the two oval pads.

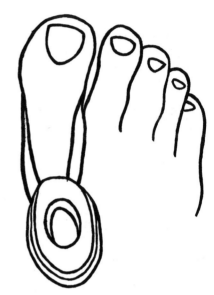

Figure 1.

6. The entire pad is now remove from the hallux and an apertur is fashioned into the oval to ac commodate the size of the le sion.
7. Taper all edges with scissors t desired fit (Fig. 1).

ADDITIONAL COMMENTS
To prolong the life of the pad, piece of moleskin of same size an shape can be adhered over the en tire pad.

PAD TO CONTROL HYPERMOBILE FIRST RAY

INDICATION

To conservatively control the hypermobile first segment while protecting lesions occurring under the first metatarsal head.

MATERIALS

1. ⅛" or ¹⁄₁₆" nonadhesive felt.
2. Spatula.
3. Liquid latex or silicone.
4. Indelible ink pen.
5. Alcohol.
6. 1" fabco gauze.
7. Micropore tape.

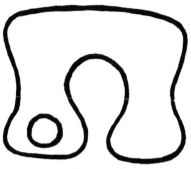

Figure 1.

BOUNDARIES

The pad extends from the plantar aspect of the first metatarsal head to the proximal phalanx of the hallux. The pad will encircle the entire area of the first metatarsophalangeal articulation.

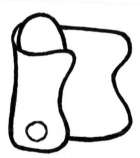

Figure 2.

CONSTRUCTION

1. Using a piece of ⅛" or ¹⁄₁₆" nonadhesive felt, fashion a shape approximately 2" × 3".
2. From this felt piece, fashion a template using Figure 1 as a guide. When finished, the template should fit over the first metatarsal phalangeal articulation as follows. Plantarly the

pad should be wide enough to cover the entire medial plantar aspect of the foot and be able to accept an aperture to accommodate any first metatarsal plantar lesions. The narrowest part of the pad will pass through the first interspace and dorsally to wrap around the entire proximal phalanx of the hallux. Be sure to leave an extra tab on the pad so that the

Polokoff, Morton M.: Orthodigita: Removable Felt and Silicone Appliances for Conservative Treatment of Hypermobility of the First Segment. *J.A.P.A.*, 64 (9), September 1974, pp. 721-729.

excess will continue to encircle the plantar surface of the proximal phalanx of the hallux (Fig. 1).

3. Now impregnate the entire pad with liquid latex or silicone using a spatula. Spread just enough silicone to impregnate the material without the latex oozing to the point where it becomes unmanageable. Allow to dry partially.

4. Mark the entire lesion beneath the first metatarsal head with an indelible pen. Place a few drops of alcohol on the template where you expect the ink marking to transfer.

5. Now wrap the template around the great toe into proper position. Be sure to transfer the marking to the template (Fig. 2).

6. With sharp scissors, cut an aperture into the template at the transfer mark to accommodate the entire circumference of the lesion.

7. Now impregnate the pad with more silicone as in step 3. Replace the pad and trim away the excess after the pad has been adjusted to fit properly over the hallux.

8. Now wrap the entire pad with 1″ fabco encircling the hallux two or three times. Be careful to wrap firmly but not too loose or too tight.

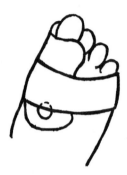

Figure 3.

9. Impregnate with silicone again.

10. Secure the pad to the foot with micropore tape until the entire construction dries (Fig. 3).

11. Cover the entire pad with a small plastic bag. The patient is instructed to wear the pad with the plastic bag in the shoe until bedtime.

12. At the next visit the molded pad can be trimmed to proper fit.

ADDITIONAL COMMENTS

1. Silicone can be added at subsequent visits to accommodate for lesion discomfort.

2. Dusting with talcum powder daily will enhance the life of the pad.

3. The pad can be washed with soap and water and left to dry overnight.

PLASTIZOTE HAV SHIELD

INDICATIONS

To construct a removable bunion pad that will relieve pressure from a painful lesion at the proximal aspect of the first metatarsal phalangeal joint.

MATERIALS

1. ⅛″ plastizote.
2. ⅛″ or ¼″ adhesive foam or adhesive felt.
3. Linen.
4. No. 2A tubegauze.
5. 1⁄16″ plastizote.
6. Heating element.
7. Rubber cement.

BOUNDARIES

The pad will extend over the entire hallux and encircle the great toe to include the medial aspect of the first metatarsal 2″ proximal to the bunion deformity.

CONSTRUCTION

1. Encircle the foot with two 1″ strips of adhesive moleskin. One strip fits around the medial aspect of the foot about 2½″ proximal to the first metatarsal phalangeal joint. The second strip is placed directly over the first metatarsal phalangeal joint.

McDonald, R.: Hand Moulded Plastizote Appliances, *The Chiropodist*, July 1967, pp. 235-239.

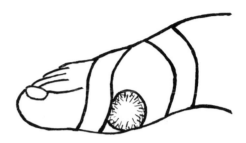

Figure 1.

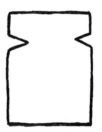

Figure 2.

2. The first metatarsal phalangeal joint may also require a deep pocket for construction of the finished shield. Therefore, you may cut a ⅛″ adhesive felt circle of 1″ diameter which can then be adhered to the bunion excrescence directly (Fig. 1).
3. Now cut a section of ⅛″ plastizote into a 6″ × 4″ sheet and then fashion the sheet according to the dimensions in Figure 2. The "V" shaped slits will

help to form the area from which the great toe band can be molded (Fig. 2).

4. The plastizote sheet is then heated until it is moldable.

5. Now quickly apply a small amount of adhesive to the inner ends of the 1½" flanges which were fashioned in Step 3 (Fig. 3).

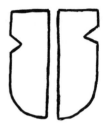

Figure 3.

6. Now place the plastizote against the great toe and medial border of the foot. The toe flanges are molded around the toe, and the adhesive coated ends are pressed firmly together. Then mold the remainder of the plastizote over the bunion and moleskin strips around the medial aspect of the foot. This should be done quickly as the plastizote cools within a short time (Fig. 4).

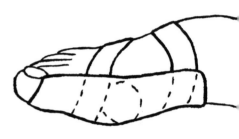

Figure 4.

7. Now apply adhesive over the entire area of the plastizote mold while it remains on the foot.

8. Fashion a crescent pad of adhesive felt or adhesive foam of desired depth according to the guidelines outlined on page 68.

9. Adhere the crescent to the plastizote mold at the medial proximal aspect of the excrescence created by the bunion (Fig. 5).

10. The outer surface of the crescent is then coated with spray adhesive.

11. Fashion two pieces of linen according to the measurements in Figure 4.

12. Now place the two strips of lin-

en over the pad about ½" apart allowing the flanges to once again encircle the great toe.

13. Coat the linen strips with spray adhesive.

14. Cut the lateral aspect of the plastizote toe section along its long axis leaving a ¼" opening of exposed skin surface.

15. Cut a 1" length of No. 2A surgitube to encircle the entire hallux.

16. Coat the surgitube toe net with adhesive on all sides and slip the tube over the plastizote which is on the hallux.

17. Now a second piece of plastizote the same size and shape as

the first layer is heated and molded over the entire pad being sure to include the toe loop (Fig. 6).

18. After the entire pad has cooled, remove the appliance from the foot. The moleskin and felt dome are now removed from the foot and discarded. The shield is now trimmed to shape.

19. The edges of the shield can be reduced to a fine, sealed border by first skiving the edges, then heating the rim of the appliance over a flame at approximately a 6″ distance. Then roll the hot edges over a flat surface. Take care when heating the plastizote as it may brown if too close to the flame.

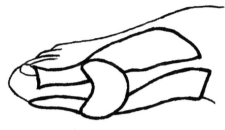

Figure 5.

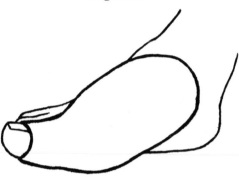

Figure 6.

POLOKOFF HALLUX SHIELD

INDICATIONS
To construct a long-lasting removable shield for inflamed bunions, lesions under the hallux, lesions under the first metatarsal
head, hallux rigidus or heloma molle between the first and second
toes.

Figure 1.

MATERIALS
1. No. 2A tubegauze.
2. Rubber cement.
3. Liquid latex.
4. Talcum powder.
5. Felt pads of varying thickness.
6. Scissors.
7. Air blower.
8. ½" elastoplast.

BOUNDARIES
The pad covers the entire hallux
and extends proximally to midshaft of the first metatarsal covering the dorsal, medial and plantar
aspect of the foot.

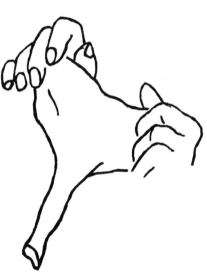

Figure 2.

CONSTRUCTION
1. Cut an 11" length of No. 2A
   tubegauze.
2. Slit the tubegauze from one
   end leaving about 4" uncut
   (Fig. 1).
3. Stretch out the slit portion to
   obtain more width (Fig. 2).

Polokoff, Morton Meyer: The Polokoff Hallux
Shield. *J.A.P.A.*, 60 (12), December 1970, pp.
480-483.

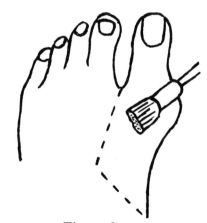

Figure 3.

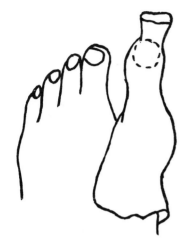

Figure 4.

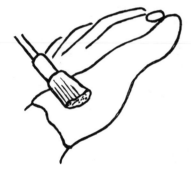

Figure 5.

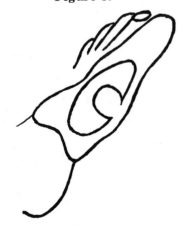

Figure 6.

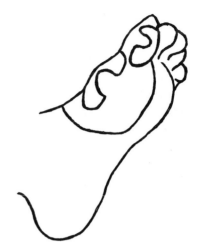

Figure 7.

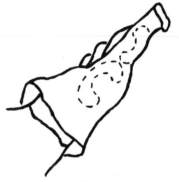

Figure 8.

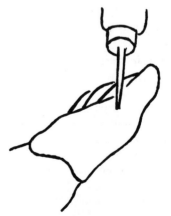

Figure 9.

4. Brush rubber cement on the skin area to be covered by the appliance (Fig. 3).

5. Turn the tubegauze inside out and pull the closed end over the hallux and draw it down to the first webspace (Fig. 4).

6. Apply rubber cement to the edges of the tubegauze and cement the tube to the skin (Fig. 5).

7. Fold the distal end of the tubegauze plantarly under the hallux to close off the end of the tubegauze (Fig. 6).

8. Brush a heavy layer of rubber cement on to the tubegauze.

9. Use "C" shaped aperture pads consisting of adhesive felt of varying thicknesses to encircle any lesions located under the tubegauze (Fig. 7).

10. Cut another 11″ length tubegauze exactly as the first and fit over the appliance. Only apply cement to the edges on the undersurface of this tubegauze for adhesion (Fig. 8).

11. Without tension, close off the distal end of the second tubegauze layer as described in Step 7.

12. Apply a generous layer of liquid latex to the entire appliance (Fig. 9).

13. If necessary, apply a second layer of liquid latex to give more support to the shield.

14. Place the entire foot in a plastic bag and instruct the patient to wear the pad in the shoe until the pad dries.

15. At the next visit, the edges of

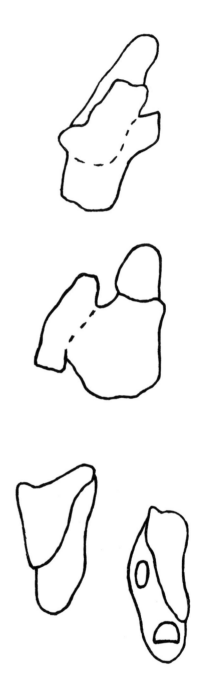

Figure 10.

the shield can be trimmed to fit
(Fig. 10).

ADDITIONAL COMMENTS

1. To afford better comfort, line the interior of the shield with adhesive moleskin. Spare the toe section and trim to the contours of the shield.

2. When the felt pads compress due to wear, additional pads may be adhered to the shield.
3. The shield can be cut to allow for painful club nails.
4. Holes may also be punctured into the appliance to afford better air circulation.

WEIGHT-BEARING LATEX BUNION SHIELD

INDICATIONS
To construct a removable long-lasting shield for bunion discomfort.

MATERIALS
1. Eight 6″ × 1″ fast drying plaster splints.
2. Skin marker.
3. Fast drying plaster.
4. Liquid latex.
5. Buildup material (corex, leather, plastizote, etc.).
6. 6″ wooden stick.
7. Sandpaper.

BOUNDARIES
This shield will encircle the entire hallux from its distal aspect and extend proximally to cover the entire painful bunion deformity.

CONSTRUCTION
1. With a skin marker outline the entire area that is painful by drawing a circle around the bunion.
2. The prepared 6″ × 1″ plaster splints are then individually immersed into lukewarm water and applied to the medial aspect of the foot. The splints will entirely encircle the hallux forming a cast that extends

Dowdeswell-Childs, T.G.: Replaceable Padding for Geriatrics. *The Chiropodist*, 21 (1), January 1968, pp. 33-37.

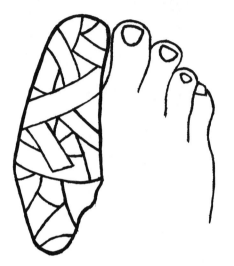

Figure 1.

proximally to include and cover the entire bunion (Fig. 1).
3. Before the plaster splints dry, the patient is instructed to assume a relaxed weight-bearing position.
4. After the cast has dried, it is removed from the foot and then filled with plaster to produce a positive impression of the area to be treated (Fig. 2).
5. Before the plaster positive is completely dry, a stay prop should be inserted into the drying plaster. This will allow easier handling when dipping the cast into the liquid latex (Fig. 3).
6. After the positive has completely dried, strip the plaster

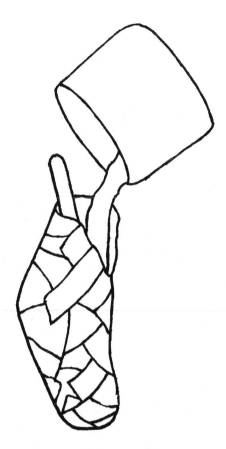

Figure 2.

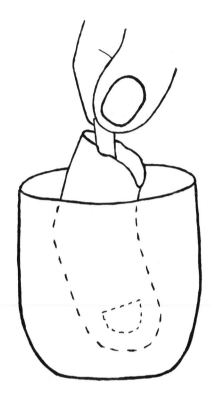

Figure 3.

splints from the mold. Smooth all rough spots by lightly sanding the impression while wetting the roughened areas with water.

7. Holding the stay prop stick gently, submerge the plaster positive into liquid latex. The cast is then stabilized on the stay prop to allow for even drying and all excess latex to drip off.

8. The cast is set aside to dry for one hour after which the sub-

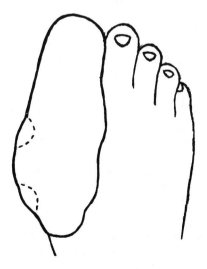

Figure 4.

merging procedure is repeated. Be sure all air bubbles are punctured immediately so that a smooth latex surface is maintained.

9. After the second coat has completely dried, buildup material of choice may be adhered to the latex shield with the purpose of removing pressure from the desired areas (Fig. 4).

10. The entire shield is then submerged into the latex one or two more times. This procedure will incorporate the buildup material into the shield and also will ensure a smooth surface and added strength to the shield.

11. When thorougly dry, remove the shield from the cast. Then scissor cut the latex form to desired shape and fit. Dust with talcum powder and apply to the foot.

ADDITIONAL COMMENTS

1. This shield will last indefinitely if it is occasionally dusted with talcum powder.

2. If excessive perspiration exists, holes may be punctured into the shield with a straight pin at desired areas.

A LEATHER REMOVABLE BUNION SHIELD

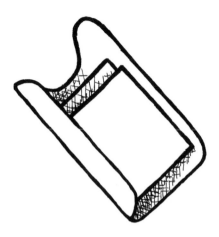

INDICATIONS
To prevent pressure and friction due to painful bunion deformity.

MATERIALS
1. 2″ × 3″ thin glazed leather.
2. Broom handle.
3. Adhesive felt or adhesive foam of desired thickness.
4. Spray adhesive.

BOUNDARIES
The medial aspect of the foot from a point immediately proximal to the excrescence to a point 3″ proximally along the first metatarsal shaft.

CONSTRUCTION
1. Cut a piece of thin glazed leather 2″ × 3″.
2. Skive the rough edges on all sides.
3. Place the leather in a glass of warm water and soak thoroughly.
4. With the glazed side up, wrap the leather around a broom handle or similar sized cylinder. The long axis of the leather should lie parallel to the long axis of the cylinder.
5. Cover the wet leather with a second piece of dry leather and strap these together on the cylinder with a piece of cord.
6. Set aside to dry. After drying, remove top leather shield.
7. You are now left with a curved leather template that can be built up as necessary with felt or adhesive foam on the concave face.
8. Adhere the appropriate foam or felt to the interior of the cylinder so that the area proximal to the bunion is buttressed. Spray foot with adhesive spray and adhere the pad directly to the skin.
9. Quickly place a stocking or sock over the pad while it is in position and wear the appliance for a few days in a shoe. This will allow the leather to shape itself to the foot.

ADDITIONAL COMMENTS
After the pad retains the proper shape it may then be worn over the sock or stocking.

Joseph, Alfred: An Ideal Bunion Shield. *Chiropody Record*, 8 (9), 1925, p. 12.

IN-SHOE BUNION SHIELDS

INDICATIONS
To relieve pain caused by pressure of the shoe against the inflamed medial aspect of the first MPJ.

MATERIALS
1. 1½" × 1¼" rectangle of ¼" corex, adhesive felt, adhesive foam.
2. ¹⁄₁₆" kid leather.

BOUNDARIES
The pad is placed immediately proximal to the bunion on the medial aspect of the shoe.

CONSTRUCTION
1. Shape the rectangle of corex, felt or foam into a crescent as described on page 68.
2. The concave portion of the pad is then placed into the shoe just proximal to the small pocket created in the shoe vamp by the bunion. If there is no pocket, the bunion can be marked in the shoe by locating the lesion with a thin needle on the shoe surface while the patient is weight-bearing. After the bump is found, the patient removes the shoe and the needle is inserted through the shoe vamp. The pad may then be placed in proper position within the shoe.
3. After affixing the pad in the shoe

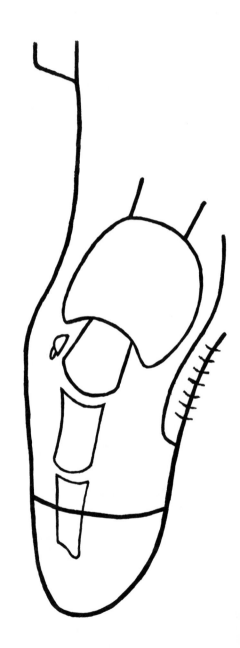

Berger, O.R.: Shoe Padding for Bunions, Tailor's Bunions and Heloma Dura. *Chiropody Record*, 28 (2), February 1945, pp. 17-20.

with rubber cement, the leather cover is then cemented over the pad and set aside to dry.

ADDITIONAL COMMENTS
If the shoe is fully leather lined, the inside surface of the shoe should be roughened with fine sandpaper before the pad is adhered.

THE VOLCANO PAD

INDICATIONS
Reduction of shoe pressure over any excrescence of the foot.

MATERIALS
1. 2″ piece of moleskin.
2. Curved scissors.
3. Spray adhesive.

BOUNDARIES
Encircling the entire painful area around the excrescence.

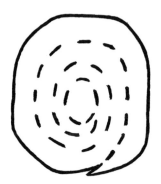

Figure 1.

CONSTRUCTION
1. Leaving the protective backing on the adhesive moleskin, cut a 2″ × 2″ square.
2. Round the edges of the square to obtain a circle with a 2″ diameter.
3. Cut the moleskin, following the circumference of the circle, gradually cutting toward its center; this procedure will produce a coil of moleskin approximately ¼″ wide, with a "pig's tail" configuration (Fig. 1).
4. Remove the protective adhesive backing of the moleskin and prepare the area to be treated with spray adhesive.
5. Apply the moleskin to the excrescence, adhering the central end of coil over the central area of the lesion.
6. Wind the coil around the lesion from its apex to its base, leav-

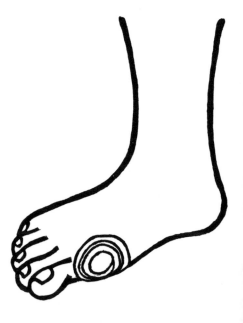

Figure 2.

ing an $\frac{1}{8}$" overlap for each successive wrap.

7. The finished coil should leave a $\frac{1}{4}$" diameter bare spot at the apex of the lesion to allow for any swelling (Fig. 2).

8. The pad is then finished by adhering a second piece of moleskin (3" diameter) over the volcano pad.

"T" SLING FOR HALLUX VALGUS

INDICATIONS
To remove pressure from a painful second toe that is being caused by a flexible hallux valgus deformity.

MATERIALS
1. 3" moleskin.
2. Straight scissors.

BOUNDARIES
The moleskin will encircle the base of the hallux and extend proximally where it is secured on the medial aspect of the first metatarsal shaft.

CONSTRUCTION
1. Using sharp straight scissors, cut the 3" moleskin into a "T" shape so that the horizontal bar of the "T" is 1" wide by 2½" long and the vertical bar of the "T" is 1" wide by 4" long (Fig. 1).
2. Prepare the first metatarsal and hallux by spraying with adhesive.
3. Wrap the 2½" horizontal bar around the base of the hallux leaving the vertical bar directly over the medial aspect of the first MPJ. The vertical bar will point in a proximal direction.
4. Now passively adduct the hallux until it is articulating with the first metatarsal head and the valgus deformity is corrected.
5. While holding the great toe in corrected position, adhere the

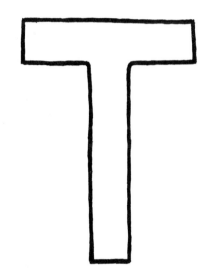

Figure 1.

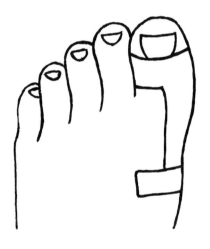

Figure 2.

vertical member of the "T" tightly to the medial aspect of the first metatarsal head and shaft.

6. Secure the vertical bar with 1″ adhesive tape where necessary (Fig. 2).

VI
LESSER TOES

Aperture Pad or U-Pad for
Lesser Toes

Removable Sling for
Underlapping Lesser Toe

Removable Felt Hammer Toe
Pad

Temporary Removable
Buttress Appliance (Crest
Pad)

Removable Felt Toe Traction
Pad

Dynamically Molded
Temporary Removable
Buttress Appliance

Dressing for Extensive Heloma
Durum

Removable Digital Pad

Removable Latex Sponge
Heloma Durum Shield

Removable Latex Sponge
Plantar Prop

Removable Latex Hammer Toe
or Lesser Toe Shield

Removable Hammer Toe Pad
with Protective Flap for
Distal Excrescence

Removable Latex Lesser Toe
Splint

Removable Double Cotton Roll
Buttress ·

Latex Lesser Toe Replacement
Device

Removable Latex Distal
Heloma Shield

Felt Under Pad

Heloma Molle Padding with
Transverse Pedis Strapping

Removable Latex Heloma
Molle Appliance

Polyurethane Foam Heloma
Molle Pads

Nail Inversion Pad

Felt Traction Appliance for
Second Toe

Felt Orthodigital Traction Pad
for Third Toe

Removable Traction Appliance
for Third Toe

Removable Traction Appliance
for Fourth Toe

Dorsal Tendon Pad

Removable Latex Fifth Toe
Heloma Durum Shield Made
with Tubular Gauze

Removable Device for Fifth
Metatarsal Head Lesions

Removable Polyurethane
Appliances

Butterfly Strapping for Nail
Inversion

APERTURE PAD OR U-PAD FOR LESSER TOES

INDICATIONS
Aperture pad: to relieve the symptoms of heloma durum.

U-pad: to relieve the pressure on soft-tissue lesions or heloma durum.

MATERIALS
$\frac{1}{16}''$, $\frac{1}{8}''$, $\frac{1}{4}''$, or $\frac{1}{2}''$ adhesive or non-adhesive felt, chamois, moleskin, sponge rubber, scissors, rubber cement.

BOUNDARIES
The pad is placed about the area in an attempt to distribute pressure away from the lesion, bone, and joint involved.

CONSTRUCTION
1. Select an appropriate material of suitable thickness; do not make the pad too thick.
2. Cut the material to approximate the size of the entire area to be shielded.
3. Fold the material in half along its long axis (do not approximate the adhesive sides of any adhesive material).
4. Cut an aperture or U that will, when fitted, just surround the lesion; the pad should not touch the lesion or be too large; posi-

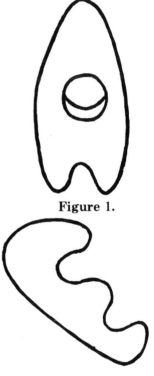

Figure 1.

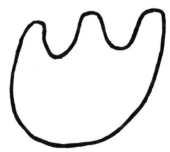

Figure 2.

Figure 3.

tion the aperture in the center of the distal half of the material, insuring that the bulk of the padding will be proximal to the lesion (Fig. 1).

5. Trim the pad to the configuration that best fits the area around the lesion; shapes commonly utilized include oval, circular, tear-drop, horse-shoe, crescent, and others (Figs. 2-5).

6. Skive the pad to feather edges; the greatest thickness should remain just about the lesion and proximal to it.

7. Adhere pad to toe; use rubber cement if material is non-adhesive.

8. Bind pad to toe using Elastoplast, podiatry tape, Gaustex, lamb's wool, or other suitable material.

ADDITIONAL COMMENTS

A suitable medication can be applied to the lesion within the aper-

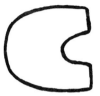

Figure 4.

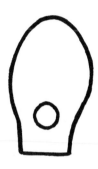

Figure 5.

ture and covered with a plug of sterile cotton before the padding is secured with a binding.

REMOVABLE SLING FOR UNDERLAPPING LESSER TOE

INDICATIONS
To correct underlapping lesser toe.

MATERIALS
Elastoplast or rubber dam, rubber cement, scissors.

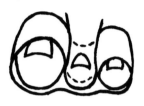

BOUNDARIES
For underlapping second toe, the sling will encircle the first and third toes while cradling the second toe. For underlapping third toe, the sling will encircle the second and fourth toes while cradling the third. For underlapping fourth toe, the sling will encircle the third and fifth toes while cradling the fourth toe.

CONSTRUCTION
For underlapping second toe:
1. Loop a ¾" or 1" wide length of Elastoplast or rubber dam over the first toe (from medial to lateral), down into the first interdigital space, under the second toe, up into the second interdigital space, over the third toe (from medial to lateral), and down into the third interdigital space.
2. Bring the strip back medially under the third, second, and first toes and up around the medial aspect of the hallux.
3. Overlap and adhere the ends together on the medial side of the first toe.
4. Examine fit to ensure that sling does not cut into web space tissue.

Similar steps may be taken to construct the sling for underlapping third or fourth toes. Start the loop over the toe medial to the involved one.

ADDITIONAL COMMENTS
The double thickness beneath the underlapping digit encourages its dorsal displacement. A plug of ⅛" or ¼" adhesive felt can be incorporated between these layers to further encourage correction.

REMOVABLE FELT HAMMER TOE PAD

INDICATIONS
To help relieve the symptoms of hammer digit syndrome with dorsal or distal excrescence.

MATERIALS
³⁄₁₆" felt, Elastoplast, scissors.

BOUNDARIES
The prop of the pad is worn under the affected toe in sulcus area and the sling is worn over the digit.

CONSTRUCTION
1. Cut a 1" × 3" rectangle of ³⁄₁₆" felt.
2. Fold the top half of the felt strip upon itself and prop the now double-thickness felt under the affected toe (Fig. 1).
3. Cut the excess length of the felt strip away, leaving the folded prop.
4. Cut a 1¼" × 3½" rectangle of Elastoplast.
5. Place the folded felt prop in the middle of the length of the Elastoplast rectange, on the adhesive surface (Fig. 2).
6. Fold the Elastoplast over the felt prop, approximating the adhesive surfaces, thereby encasing the felt completely.
7. Cut a hole in the Elastoplast

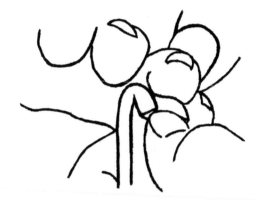

Figure 1.

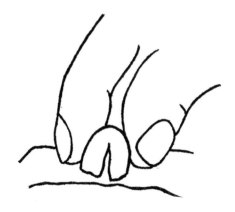

Figure 2.

Polokoff, M.M.: *Australian Podiatrist*, 10 (1), 1976, p. 74.

flap just large enough to admit the affected toe.

8. Place the toe through the sling and adjust pad on the toe so that the prop is positioned under the toe into the sulcus.

9. Trim any excess Elastoplast, rounding the edges of the sling (Fig. 3).

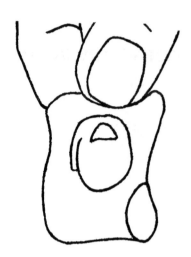

Figure 3.

TEMPORARY REMOVABLE BUTTRESS APPLIANCE
(CREST PAD)

INDICATIONS
To help correct contracted lesser digits; to help relieve the pressure on lesions associated with these.

MATERIALS
¼" or ½" diameter dental cotton roll, 3" Elastoplast, scissors.

BOUNDARIES
The sling is worn over the affected toes with the buttress under the same digits in the sulcus area.

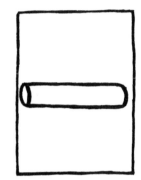

Figure 1.

CONSTRUCTION
1. Choose the appropriate size cotton roll by examination of the patient.
2. Cut a length of cotton to span the width of the affected toes (1, 2, 3 or 4 digits may be treated with this appliance; the hallux should not be included in this treatment); trim the ends so that no irritation to adjacent toes occurs.
3. Cut a length of Elastoplast that is as wide as the width of the cotton roll.
4. Place the cotton roll on the adhesive surface of the Elastoplast midway along the length of the Elastoplast rectangle (Fig. 1).
5. Fold the Elastoplast over the

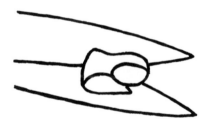

Figure 2.

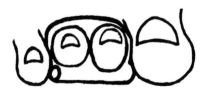

Figure 3.

Polokoff, M.M.: *J.A.P.A.*, 64 (10), 1974, p. 798.

cotton roll, approximating the adhesive surfaces, completely encasing the cotton roll.

6. Fold the now double-thickness Elastoplast flap extending from the cotton roll in half upon itself (Fig. 2).

7. Make a cut through this fold up to the edge of the cotton roll but not into the cotton roll; place the cut so that it corresponds to the center of each affected digit over which the pad will be worn.

8. Place the affected toes through the corresponding cuts in the Elastoplast flap and adjust th pad so that the cotton roll but tress is in place under the digit in the sulcus.

9. Trim the appliance and adjus to patient comfort; round edge of the sling (Fig. 3).

ADDITIONAL COMMENTS

Subsequently, build-ups of th appropriate thickness of adhesiv felt may be added to the surface c the cotton roll directly beneath th toes to enhance the extension of th toes upon ambulation.

REMOVABLE FELT TOE TRACTION PAD

INDICATIONS
To relieve the symptoms of heloma durum, heloma molle, or distal heloma and to correct contracted or malaligned lesser toes.

MATERIALS
$\frac{1}{16}''$ 90% wool-10% cotton felt, rubber cement, scissors.

BOUNDARIES
The pad is worn over the desired toes with a rolled flap propped in the sulcus under the lesser digits.

CONSTRUCTION
1. Cut a 4″ × 6″ felt square.
2. Fold one edge of the square 1″ back upon itself.
3. Cut openings in this folded section slightly smaller than the thickness of the toes over which the pad will be worn.
4. Work the felt over the toes with the long flap extending onto the plantar surface of the foot; round off all edges.
5. Contour that section of the plantar flap under the first metatarsal head and part (or all) of that section under the fifth metatarsal head (Fig. 1).
6. Paint rubber cement on the surface of the plantar flap that approximates the plantar surface of the foot; allow cement to dry.
7. Roll the flap tightly onto itself up into the sulcus under the middle three digits (Fig. 2).

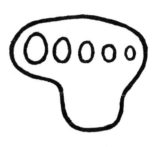

Figure 1.

ADDITIONAL COMMENTS
The pad should be worn continuously. Buildups can be added, as warranted, to both plantar and dorsal aspects of the pad.

Original contribution: Bluhm, L.W., *Journal of the National Association of Chiropodists*, 41, (6), 1951, p. 23.

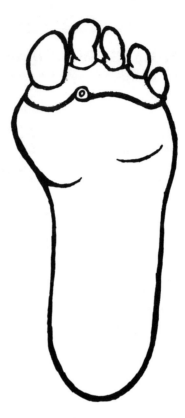

Figure 2.

DYNAMICALLY MOLDED TEMPORARY REMOVABLE BUTTRESS APPLIANCE

INDICATIONS

To help correct contracted or hammered lesser toes; to help relieve the pressure on dorsal or distal lesions associated with these; to help force anteriorly displaced soft tissue back under the metatarsal heads.

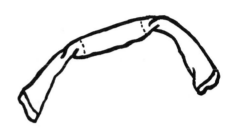

Figure 1.

MATERIALS

No. 1 Surgitube, ¼″ or ½″ diameter dental cotton roll, adhesive moleskin, rubber cement, liquid latex, scissors, powder.

BOUNDARIES

The prop of the pad is worn under the 2nd, 3rd, and 4th toes in the sulcus area while the sling is worn over the same digits.

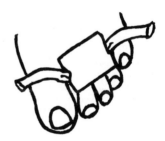

Figure 2.

CONSTRUCTION

1. Cut a 6″ length of No. 1 Surgitube.
2. Choose the appropriate size dental roll by examination of the patient.
3. Cut a length of cotton roll to span the width of the sulcus beneath the 2nd, 3rd, and 4th toes; trim the ends so that no irritation to the 1st or 5th toes occurs.
4. Slide the scissors completely

olokoff, M.M., *Chiropody Record*, 39 (1),)56, pp. 2, 6.

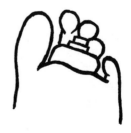

Figure 3.

through the length of Surgitube so that the tips of the
blades are visible; grasp the
end of the cotton roll with the
blades and draw the cotton roll
half-way into the Surgitube
and release it there; withdraw
the scissors through the remaining length of the Surgitube (Fig. 1).

5. Press the now encased cotton
   roll into the sulcus area under
   the middle three digits.

6. Bring the loose ends of the
   Surgitube up through the 1st
   and 4th interdigital spaces.

7. Cut a square of moleskin the
   width of which measures the
   distance from the medial border of the 2nd digit to the lateral border of the 4th digit (Fig.
   2).

8. Cut a small pie-wedge shaped
   notch in the center of each
   lateral edge of the moleskin.

9. Apply a ½-inch wide strip of
   rubber cement to the non-adhesive surface of the moleskin
   spanning the distance between
   the notches.

10. Apply a ½-inch wide strip of
    rubber cement to the dorsal
    surfaces of the proximal pha-
    langes of the 2nd, 3rd, and 4th
    toes.

11. Adhere the moleskin square to
    the dorsum of the digits by ap-
    proximating the rubber ce-
    ment coated surfaces of the
    moleskin and patient's skin.

12. Adhere the loose end of th
    Surgitube in the 1st interspac
    onto the adhesive surface of th
    moleskin, which is now facin
    up; the Surgitube end shoul
    pass through the notch tha
    was cut in the moleskin edg
    trim any excess length of Surg
    tube.

13. Adhere the loose end of Surg
    tube in the 4th interspace in
    similar manner.

14. Fold the distal and proxima
    flaps of moleskin, respectively
    onto the now adhered ends c
    Surgitube, firmly securin
    them in place on the dorsum

15. Apply liquid latex to the entir
    appliance, including the Surg
    tube in the interdigital space
    while in place on the patient
    foot.

16. Dry the device carefully with
    hot air blower for 5 to 10 mir
    utes; powder the appliance be
    fore replacing hose; if device
    still damp, cover with pap
    toweling or other suitable ma
    terial before replacing hose.

ADDITIONAL COMMENTS

The appliance should be worn ur
til the affected toes have acquire
near normal position; 3 to
months of continuous wear may k
required. Additional felt or mol
skin build-ups can be adhered t
either the buttress or dorsal areas
the device as necessary (Fig. 3).

DRESSING FOR EXTENSIVE HELOMA DURUM

INDICATIONS
To dress a lesser digit heloma durum which extends across the entire width of the toe and which cannot be shielded by conventional felt padding.

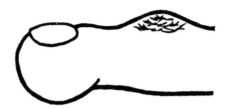

Figure 1.

MATERIALS
Absorbent cotton, spray or liquid adhesive, adhesive tape, medicated ointment, scissors.

BOUNDARIES
The dressing is applied to the affected area of the dorsum of the digit.

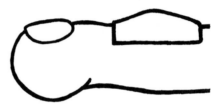

Figure 2.

CONSTRUCTION
1. Debride the lesion by accepted means.
2. Apply a medicated ointment of choice over the lesion (Fig. 1).
3. Spray or apply adhesive to the remainder of the toe, not over the lesion.
4. Cover the lesion and adhesive-coated surface of toe with a thin layer of absorbent cotton.
5. Cut a strip of adhesive tape which measures as wide as the

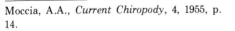

Moccia, A.A., *Current Chiropody*, 4, 1955, p. 14.

dorsum of the toe and as long as the area to be covered.
6. Adhere the tape in place on the dorsum of the toe so that it covers the cotton dressing completely and adheres to the skin just surrounding the dressing (Fig. 2).
7. Anchor the dressing onto the toe with $\frac{1}{8}''$ wide adhesive tape, self-adhering gauze, or a few turns of lamb's wool.

REMOVABLE DIGITAL PAD

INDICATIONS
To help relieve the symptoms of heloma durum affecting a lesser digit.

MATERIALS
$\frac{1}{32}$" or $\frac{1}{16}$" non-adhesive felt, $\frac{1}{8}$" or $\frac{1}{4}$" adhesive felt, adhesive moleskin, scissors.

BOUNDARIES
The body of the pad sits on the dorsum of the affected toe while the digit itself is positioned through a plantar loop.

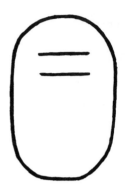

Figure 1.

CONSTRUCTION
1. Cut a rectangle of non-adhesive felt 1½" wide and 2" in length.
2. Make two cuts, ¼" apart, perpendicular to the length of the felt rectangle; the first cut should be ½" from the distal edge of the rectangle and the second should be ¾" from the same edge; each cut should be 1" in length (Fig. 1).
3. Fashion a suitable U-pad from adhesive felt to accommodate the dorsal lesion.
4. Place the non-adhesive felt rectangle onto the affected toe by sliding the digit through the plantar loop fashioned above in Step 2.
5. Adhere the adhesive felt U-pad

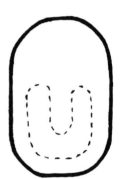

Figure 2.

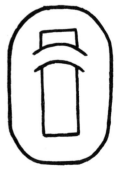

Original contribution by E.E. Sugarman.

Figure 3.

onto the portion of the non-adhesive felt rectangle that now lies on the dorsum of the toe; position it to shield the lesion on the digit, with the bulk of the pad proximal to the excrescence.

6. Cover the entire dorsal surface of the resultant two-layer pad with a rectangle of adhesive moleskin, thereby sandwiching the adhesive U-pad between the non-adhesive felt rectangle and this adhesive moleskin layer; press edges down firmly (Fig. 2).

7. Remove the pad from the patient's toe; turn it over, visualizing the plantar aspect and the loop; cut a strip of adhesive moleskin 1″ wide and 1½″ long and adhere it beneath the plantar loop so as to cover the rectangular defect created in the non-adhesive felt while fashioning the loop in Step 2; the adhesive surface of this moleskin strip should contact the felt pad and not the skin of the patient's toe (Fig. 3).

8. Round the edges of the pad and fit to the patient's foot.

REMOVABLE LATEX SPONGE HELOMA DURUM SHIELD

INDICATIONS
To help relieve the symptoms of heloma durum affecting a lesser digit.

MATERIALS
³⁄₁₆″ adhesive latex sponge, rubber sheeting, adhesive moleskin, scissors.

BOUNDARIES
The body of the shield sits on the dorsum of the affected digit while the toe itself is positioned through the plantar loop.

CONSTRUCTION
1. Cut a tear-drop shaped shield from ³⁄₁₆″ adhesive latex sponge, approximately 1½″ to 2″ long and ¾″ to 1″ wide, with the widest part of the tear-drop distal.
2. Cut a suitable aperture that will accommodate the lesion.
3. Position the shield on the affected toe, aperture about the lesion, with the nonadhesive surface of the sponge on the skin.

Drew, F.A., *British Journal of Chiropody*, 20 (1), 1955, p. 13.

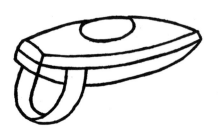

4. Cut a ⅓″ × 4″ length of rubber sheeting and loop it around the plantar portion of the toe and onto the adhesive surface of the latex sponge shield, distal to the aperture; trim any excess length.
5. Cover the exposed adhesive surface of the latex sponge with a piece of moleskin with an aperture to match that in the latex; the adhesive surfaces of the two materials are approximated, thereby securing the rubber loop in place between the layers.
6. Trim device and fit to patient.

ADDITIONAL COMMENTS
If a thicker shield is required, the cover piece can be cut from ¹⁄₁₆″ to ³⁄₁₆″ adhesive materials. A proximal binding loop can easily be incorporated to enhance stability.

REMOVABLE LATEX SPONGE PLANTAR PROP

INDICATIONS
To help correct a contracted lesser digit.

MATERIALS
³⁄₁₆″ adhesive latex sponge, rubber sheeting, scissors.

BOUNDARIES
The body of the pad is propped under the length of the affected toe with the digit itself positioned through a dorsal loop.

CONSTRUCTION
1. Cut a strip of latex sponge that is twice the length of the affected digit and slightly wider than its width.
2. Press the latex sponge strip up under the entire length of the affected toe with the adhesive surface of the material directed plantarly away from the skin; the excess length of the strip should extend proximally away from the sulcus onto the plantar surface of the foot.

Drew, F.A., *British Journal of Chiropody*, 20 (1), 1955, p. 13.

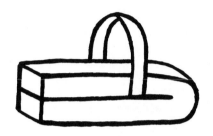

3. Cut a ⅓″ × 4″ length of rubber sheeting and loop it over the top of the digit and adhere the free ends under the digit onto the adhesive surface of the latex sponge, in the proximal third of the length of the strip under the toe, so that the loop will lie over the proximal phalanx; trim any excess length.
4. Check the tension of the loop; bring the proximal half of the latex strip, by folding, to meet the distal half, approximating the adhesive surfaces and thereby securing the rubber loop in place between the two layers.
5. Trim any excess material, especially at the distal extent of the prop.

REMOVABLE LATEX HAMMER TOE OR LESSER TOE SHIELD

INDICATIONS
To help relieve the symptoms of heloma durum affecting a lesser digit.

MATERIALS
Latex kit, ⅛" or ¼" sponge rubber, rubber cement, scissors.

BOUNDARIES
The shield is worn over the entire digit.

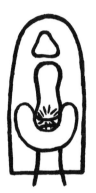

Figure 1.

CONSTRUCTION
1. Mark the excrescence (do not reduce) and the depth of the web space with an indelible marker.
2. Using accepted methods, make a negative cast of the affected digit ensuring that the plaster extends well beyond the proximal limits of the toe (i.e., onto the plantar and dorsal aspects of the foot and well into the web spaces surrounding the digit).
3. Utilizing accepted methods, make positive cast of affected digit and apply 3 layers of latex.
4. Fashion a sponge rubber (or other suitable material) aperture or U-pad to accommodate the lesion.
5. Adhere the aperture pad to the

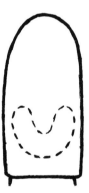

Figure 2.

latex layers on the positive cast; position the pad slightly proximal to the lesion (Fig. 1).
6. Apply 8 to 12 additional layers of latex.
7. Fit on patient and trim as necessary; ensure that the device does not "cut" into web tissue (Fig. 2).

Block, I.H., *Current Chiropody*, 5 (9), 1956, p. 9.

REMOVABLE HAMMER TOE PAD WITH PROTECTIVE FLAP FOR DISTAL EXCRESCENCE

INDICATIONS

To help relieve the pressure on both the heloma durum and distal heloma of a hammered digit.

MATERIALS

Felt or sponge rubber, of suitable thickness, 1½" wide adhesive tape, adhesive moleskin, or chamois, rubber cement (if chamois is used), scissors.

BOUNDARIES

The pad sits on the dorsum of the affected toe, with the grooved portion directed distally and the protective flap extending under the distal aspect of the digit.

CONSTRUCTION

1. Fashion a protective pad of felt or sponge rubber to accommodate the heloma durum; the pad should have a concave surface (to shield the lesion itself) and be trimmed to present a convex surface (Fig. 1).
2. Cut a 6" long strip of 1½" wide tape, moleskin, or chamois (coated with rubber cement on one surface); place the pad onto the adhesive surface of the strip with the convex surface of the

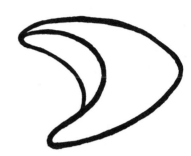

Figure 1.

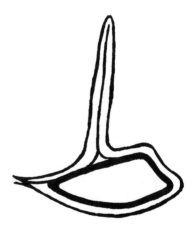

Figure 2.

pad contacting the adhesive and the proximal end of the pad ½" from the edge of the strip.

3. Work the adhesive onto the concave surface of the pad, embedding only the distal half of the shield into the strip; press down, seal, and smooth all contacting

Koppe, W.P., *Clinical Journal of Chiropody, Podiatry and Pedic Surgery*, 5 (10), 1933, p. 329.

surfaces; approximately ⅔ of the length of the strip should remain unused.

4. Fold the remaining adhesive upon itself (adhesive surface to adhesive surface), fashioning the flap, making certain to leave enough length of adhesive to fasten onto the proximal half of the pad.

5. Press down, seal, and smooth the adhesive strip onto the remaining exposed proximal portion of the shield; make certain to work the adhesive well onto all contours; trim the edges fairly close (Fig. 2).

6. Cut a U-shaped opening in the flap, with the curve of the U directed toward the body of the pad; the opening should be just large enough to admit the digit (Fig. 3).

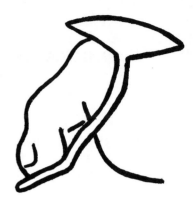

Figure 3.

ADDITIONAL COMMENTS

This device, when fashioned and worn properly, offers traction to the contracted digit and is mildly corrective.

REMOVABLE LATEX LESSER TOE SPLINT

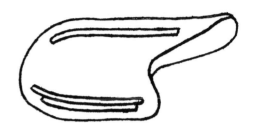

INDICATIONS

To help in the correction of a single malpositioned toe, to help train the toe into better alignment.

MATERIALS

Latex kit, $\frac{1}{16}$" rubber sheeting, $\frac{1}{16}$" leather, rubber cement, scissors.

BOUNDARIES

The device is worn over the entire digit.

CONSTRUCTION

1. Make a negative cast of the affected toe; be certain to correct the alignment of the digit by applying gentle pressure to the toe as the casting material begins to set.
2. Utilizing accepted methods, make positive cast of the affected digit and apply 3 layers of latex.
3. Adhere a strip of rubber sheeting, as wide as the toe and approximately its length, to the dorsal aspect of the latex layers on the positive cast; the strip should not lie atop the nail.
4. Adhere a similar strip of rubber sheeting along the entire plantar aspect of the latex layers on the positive cast; make certain it ends proximally well under the base of the toe.
5. Adhere a "stiffener" of $\frac{1}{16}$" leather, as wide as the toe and slightly shorter than the plantar rubber cushion, to the plantar cushion; the proximal end of the "stiffener" should be placed so that it will be cushioned by the rubber sheeting and not "cut" into the tissue at the base of the digit.
6. Apply 8 to 10 additional layers of latex.
7. Fit on patient and trim as necessary.

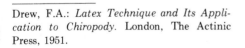

Drew, F.A.: *Latex Technique and Its Application to Chiropody.* London, The Actinic Press, 1951.

REMOVABLE DOUBLE COTTON ROLL BUTTRESS

INDICATIONS
To help relieve the symptoms of hammer digit syndrome.

MATERIALS
¼" and ½" diameter dental cotton roll, 2" wide Elastoplast, scissors.

BOUNDARIES
The device is worn over the middle three digits with a double cotton roll buttress in the sulcus area under the same toes.

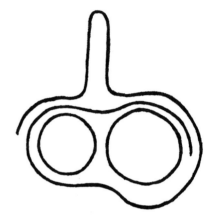

CONSTRUCTION
1. Cut a 2" length of each diameter dental cotton roll.
2. Cut a 6" length of 2" wide Elastoplast.
3. Place the ¼" diameter cotton roll on the adhesive surface of the Elastoplast 1" from one end; place the ½" diameter cotton roll next to the first, further away from the end of the strip.
4. Fold the short end of the Elastoplast over the cotton rolls so that it overlays the smaller roll and encircles halfway around the larger cotton roll.
5. The remaining end of the Elastoplast is folded over the midline between the two cotton rolls and then folded onto itself to form a dorsal tab.
6. The remaining ½" length of Elastoplast is adhered to the distal, smaller cotton roll to act as an anchor tab.
7. A suitable aperture, either a single transverse slit to accommodate all the middle digits or individual cuts for each toe, is fashioned and the device fitted to the patient's foot.

ADDITIONAL COMMENTS
The anterior roll acts as an effective prop under the distal phalanges, to help promote normal toe action and relieve pressure on the distal aspects of the digits, while the proximal roll acts as a fulcrum under the proximal interphalangeal joints.

Original contribution by Leonard Hymes.

LATEX LESSER TOE REPLACEMENT DEVICE

INDICATIONS

To replace an amputated 2nd, 3rd, or 4th digit; to help prevent or correct the deformity resulting when adjacent toe(s) move into the empty space.

MATERIALS

Latex kit, 5/16″ foam rubber, rubber cement, scissors.

BOUNDARIES

The device is worn over the adjacent toes with the foam replacement toe filling the space vacated by the amputated digit.

CONSTRUCTION

1. Using accepted methods, take a negative cast of the toes adjacent to the empty space; make certain that sufficient plaster is introduced into the space to maintain the adjacent digits in correct anatomical position; the cast should extend onto the dorsal and plantar aspects of the forefoot.
2. Make a positive cast of the affected part of the foot and apply 3 layers of latex.

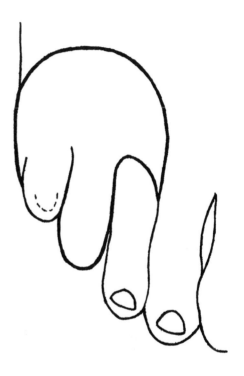

3. Fashion a replacement digit from 5/16″ foam rubber and cement it in place between the remaining toes.
4. Apply 5 to 7 additional layers of latex.
5. Fit device on patient and trim as necessary; make certain that device does not "cut" into web tissue.

Drew, F.A.: *Latex Technique and Its Application to Chiropody*. London, The Actinic Press, 1951.

REMOVABLE LATEX DISTAL HELOMA SHIELD

INDICATIONS
To help relieve the symptoms of distal heloma affecting a lesser digit.

MATERIALS
Latex kit, $\frac{1}{16}''$ or $\frac{1}{8}''$ felt, sponge rubber, leather or similar material, rubber cement, scissors.

BOUNDARIES
The device is worn over the entire digit.

CONSTRUCTION
1. Using accepted methods, make negative cast of the affected toe.
2. Make positive cast of digit and apply 3 layers of latex.
3. Fashion a "plug" $\frac{3}{8}''$ square, or sized as the case dictates, from felt, sponge rubber, leather or other suitable material; round and skive edges.

Woolf, W.: *Toe Casting and Liquid Rubber Technic*. New York, Harriman Printing Co., 1937.

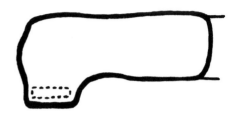

4. Adhere the "plug" to the layers of latex on the positive cast, positioning it on the plantar aspect of the distal phalanx.
5. Apply 8 to 10 additional layers of latex.
6. Fit on patient and trim as necessary.

ADDITIONAL COMMENTS
This device is most helpful in cases where no great rigidity at the distal interphalangeal joint exists and where no more than 50% of the distal plantar surface of the toe is affected by the lesion (Moon, C.L., *Current Chiropody*, 3 (11), 1953, p. 9).

FELT UNDER PAD

INDICATIONS
To relieve the symptoms of heloma molle in the fourth interdigital space or intermetatarsal neuroma in the third interdigital space.

MATERIALS
$\frac{1}{8}$" or $\frac{1}{4}$" adhesive felt, scissors.

BOUNDARIES
The pad is placed under the fourth metatarsal on the plantar surface of the foot.

CONSTRUCTION
1. Cut a piece of felt 1″ wide and as long as the entire length of the fourth metatarsal.
2. Position and adhere the strip along the length of the fourth metatarsal, from just distal to the head of the bone to its base.

ADDITIONAL COMMENTS
The pad is designed to place the heads of the third and fourth metatarsals onto different planes.

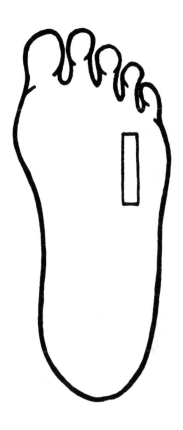

HELOMA MOLLE PADDING WITH TRANSVERSE PEDIS STRAPPING

INDICATIONS
To relieve the symptoms of heloma molle in the fourth interdigital space.

MATERIALS
1/8" or 1/4" adhesive felt, sponge rubber, rubber cement, 1" wide adhesive tape, scissors.

BOUNDARIES
The pad is placed under the third and fourth metatarsal heads; the strapping is placed as described below.

CONSTRUCTION
1. Fashion a pad approximating the length of the metatarsal shafts and shape with high point as shown (Figs. 1, 2).
2. Adhere pad to plantar surface of foot with high point under third and fourth metatarsal heads.
3. Cut an 8" length of 1" wide adhesive tape and split the last 2" of one end longitudinally.
4. Adhere the unsplit end of the tape to the dorsolateral aspect of the foot anterior to the styloid process of the fifth metatarsal; pull the tape firmly across the plantar surface and up around

Figure 1.

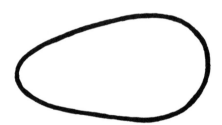

Figure 2.

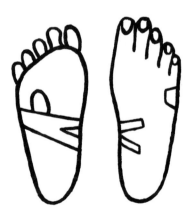

Figure 3.

Koppe, W.P., *Clinical Journal of Chiropody, Podiatry, and Pedic Surgery*, 5 (12), 1933, p. 426.

the medial aspect so that the split end of the tape terminates on the dorsum of the foot (Fig. 3).

ADDITIONAL COMMENTS

The pad is designed to raise the fourth metatarsal while the strapping maintains the fifth metatarsal in an attitude of inversion; the end result is to shift the positions of the abutting phalanges. The strapping need not touch the pad or help keep it in place.

REMOVABLE LATEX HELOMA MOLLE APPLIANCE

INDICATIONS
To help relieve the symptoms of heloma molle in any interspace.

MATERIALS
Latex kit, sponge rubber or other suitable material, rubber cement, scissors.

BOUNDARIES
The appliance is worn over the entire toe.

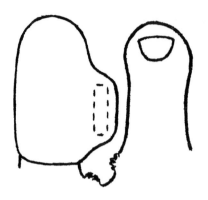

CONSTRUCTION
1. Using accepted methods, make a negative cast of the digit immediately adjacent to the digit affected with the lesion (the toe medial to the one affected if the lesion is medial or the toe lateral to the one affected if the lesion is lateral); try not to cast the digit with the lesion, unless absolutely necessary.
2. Make a positive cast of the digit and apply 3 layers of latex.
3. Fashion a separation wedge from sponge rubber or similar material that is of sufficient width to prevent the affected digit from contacting the adjacent digit.
4. Adhere this wedge to the layers of latex on the positive cast in a manner that prevents it from contacting the lesion itself.
5. Apply 5 to 7 additional layers of latex.
6. Fit on patient and trim as necessary; make certain that appliance does not "cut" into web tissue.

Snuff, E.B., *Chiropody Record*, 24, 1941, p. 3.

POLYURETHANE FOAM HELOMA MOLLE PADS

INDICATIONS

To help relieve the symptoms of heloma molle occurring in:
1. the first interspace;
2. the second, third, or fourth interspaces having distal or middle interphalangeal joint lesions;
3. any interspace having lesions near the medial nail border or in the web tissue.

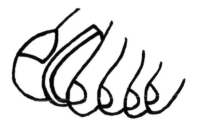

Figure 1.

MATERIALS

1" medium density polyurethane foam, scissors.

BOUNDARIES

1. Pad is worn in the 1st interspace (Fig. 1).
2. Pad is worn "cradling" either the 2nd, 3rd, or 4th toe (Fig. 2).
3. Pad is worn in the 2nd, 3rd, or 4th interspace (Fig. 3).

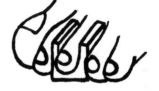

Figure 2.

CONSTRUCTION

1. The wedge (Fig. 1):

   a. Cut a piece of polyurethane foam at least ½" thick and at least as long as the 1st and 2nd digits.

   b. Round the distal aspect of the pad; cut a concave arch in the proximal end of the pad to fit into the web.

   c. Place in the 1st interspace and trim to fit patient.

2. The collar (Fig. 2):

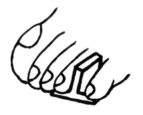

Figure 3.

Stone, J., *Current Podiatry*, 16 (1), 1967, p. 18.

a. Cut a 1″ cube of poly-urethane.

b. Cut a section, ½″ wide by ¾″ deep, from the cube; this leaves two "wings" and a central well into which the toe will be placed; remove the section so that the "wings" are of slightly varying thicknesses.

c. Place the pad on the foot so that the thicker "wing" is worn in the interspace with the lesion; the thinner "wing" is worn in the adjacent interspace while the toe is positioned in the central well.

3. The "T" pad (Fig. 3):

a. Cut a 1″ high by 1″ deep by 1¼″ long block of polyurethane foam.

b. Cut two sections from the block so that a single, centered "wing," of about ⅜″ width remains.

c. Place the pad on the foot so that the "wing" is in the affected interspace, with the adjacent toes resting on the crossbar of the "T."

ADDITIONAL COMMENTS

The thickness of the wedge (Fig. 1) can be increased to ⅝″ or ¾″ if the ½″ device does not prove successful.

NAIL INVERSION PAD

INDICATIONS

To help relieve the symptoms of onychocryptosis (nail inversion) or hypertrophied ungualabia, especially of the hallux.

MATERIALS

⅛″ or ¼″ adhesive felt, scissors, binding material.

BOUNDARIES

The pad is worn on the affected digit, covering the outer one-third of the nail plate and extending onto the side of the digit.

CONSTRUCTION

1. Cut a rectangle of ⅛″ or ¼″ adhesive felt approximately the size of the hallux nail or slightly larger.
2. Cut an aperture in the felt rectangle to accommodate the affected area of the digit; the aperture should be in the lateral half

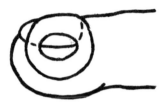

of the rectangle, off-centered to one side.
3. Adhere the lateral edge closest to the aperture onto the outer one-third of the nail plate adjacent to the affected nail fold.
4. While applying traction to the skin to relieve the pressure on the painful nail fold, adhere the remaining two-thirds of the felt pad to the side of the affected toe.
5. Bind the pad to the digit with suitable material.

ADDITIONAL COMMENTS

The aperture provides a convenient well into which a medicated ointment can be placed before binding the pad to the toe.

Koppe, W.P., *Clinical Journal of Chiropody, Podiatry and Pedic Surgery*, 6 (5), 1934, p. 155.

FELT TRACTION APPLIANCE FOR SECOND TOE

INDICATIONS
To help realign a dorsally contracted 2nd toe.

MATERIALS
⅛″ Polokoff (high wool/low cotton content) felt, scissors.

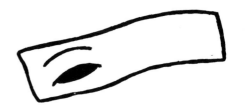

Figure 1.

BOUNDARIES
The rings of the appliance are worn over the 2nd and 4th toes with the long prop of the pad in the sulcus area beneath the 2nd, 3rd, and 4th digits.

CONSTRUCTION
1. Cut a rectangle of ⅛″ felt approximately 3½″ long by exactly 1⅛″ wide.
2. Fold over one end of the rectangle approximately one-third of its length; make 2 cuts, about ½″ long, parallel to the long axis of the rectangle exactly ⅜″ in from each edge; the loop resulting from this is about 1″ long and ⅜″ wide (Fig. 1).
3. Slip this loop over the 2nd toe and pull the toe into near normal position.
4. Fold the remaining uncut two-thirds of the felt rectangle along its long axis and press this portion into the sulcus area under

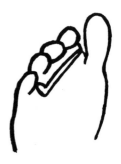

Figure 2.

the 2nd, 3rd, and 4th digits (Fig. 2).
5. Trim any excess length of felt extending beyond the 4th interdigital space.
6. Remove the device from the foot and fashion a second loop to be worn over the 4th toe; construct the loop as in Step 2, above.
7. Replace the appliance on the foot by slipping the two loops

Polokoff, M.M., *Journal of the American Podiatry Association*, 65 (1), 1975, p. 60.

over the 2nd and 4th toes (Fig. 3) and positioning the resultant double-thickness of longitudinally folded felt in the sulcus under the three middle digits.

ADDITIONAL COMMENTS

If additional traction on the 2nd toe is needed, a suitable thickness of adhesive felt, cut in the shape of an "hour-glass," can be slipped through the loop holding the 2nd toe, felt side against the skin of the dorsum of the 2nd toe, and the adhesive sides approximated (Fig. 4).

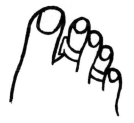

Figure 3.

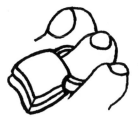

Figure 4.

FELT ORTHODIGITAL TRACTION PAD FOR THIRD TOE

INDICATIONS

To keep the third toe in proper alignment following tenotomy of the extensor tendon of that digit; to help realign a dorsally contracted third toe.

MATERIALS

³⁄₁₆″ all wool felt, scissors.

BOUNDARIES

The ring of the pad is worn over the 3rd toe with the long prop of the pad in the sulcus under the 2nd, 3rd, and 4th digits.

CONSTRUCTION

1. Cut a rectangle of ³⁄₁₆″ felt 2¼″ long by 1″ wide.
2. Fold the rectangle in half making it approximately a 1″ square.
3. Make two parallel cuts in the folded edge, ³⁄₈″ in from each edge, about ½″ long; the resulting center loop is ¼″ wide (Fig. 1).
4. Slip the loop over the third toe and fold the rectangle lengthwise so that the prop lies in the sulcus under the middle three toes.

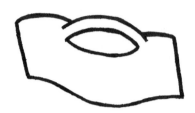

Figure 1.

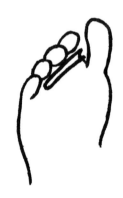

Figure 2.

5. Trim any excess length of felt that extends into the 1st or 4th interdigital spaces (Fig. 2).

ADDITIONAL COMMENTS

Following tenotomy surgery, the appliance should be worn day and night for two months to prevent tendon contracture.

Polokoff, M.M., *Journal of the National Association of Chiropodists*, 38 (5), 1948, p. 27.

REMOVABLE TRACTION APPLIANCE FOR THIRD TOE

INDICATIONS
To help realign third toe following tenotomy surgery; to help realign a dorsally contracted third toe.

MATERIALS
$\frac{1}{16}''$ or $\frac{1}{8}''$ Polokoff felt, $\frac{1}{4}''$ or $\frac{1}{2}''$ diameter dental cotton roll, rubber cement, $\frac{1}{2}''$ wide elastic adhesive, liquid latex, scissors.

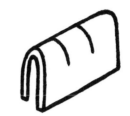

Figure 1.

BOUNDARIES
The appliance is worn over the 3rd toe, optionally over the 2nd and 4th toes, with a prop in the sulcus beneath the middle three digits.

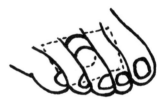

Figure 2.

CONSTRUCTION
1. Cut a $2\frac{1}{4}''$ long by $1\frac{1}{8}''$ wide rectangle of felt, $\frac{1}{8}''$ for a small foot or $\frac{1}{4}''$ for a large foot.
2. Fold the rectangle in half making it a $1\frac{1}{8}''$ square.
3. Make two parallel cuts in the folded edge, $\frac{3}{8}''$ long, $\frac{3}{8}''$ in from each edge; the resulting ring is about $\frac{3}{4}''$ long and $\frac{3}{8}''$ wide (Fig. 1).

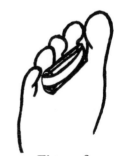

Figure 3.

4. Slip the ring over the 3rd toe and fold the rectangle lengthwise in the sulcus area under the 2nd, 3rd, and 4th digits (Fig. 2).
5. Trim any excess length of felt that extends into the 1st or 4th interdigital spaces.
6. Choose a dental cotton roll of

Polokoff, M.M., *Journal of the American Podiatry Association*, 65 (10), 1975, p. 1011.

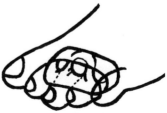

Figure 4.

appropriate diameter and cut it to the same length as the prop in the sulcus; adhere it in place into the fold of the buttress; trim any excess felt that may overlap the cotton roll plantarly.

7. Adhere one end of a ½" wide strip of elastic adhesive to the bottom of the cotton roll, near the lateral aspect of the 4th digit; adhere the strip along the entire length of the cotton roll, up through the 1st interspace, laterally over the dorsums of the 2nd, 3rd, and 4th toes, down through the 4th interspace, and back to the starting point (Fig. 3).

8. Repeat Step 7, above, so that the entire device and middle three toes have been encircled twice (Fig. 4).

9. Apply liquid latex to all elastic adhesive surfaces and to the felt; appliance should be stiff when properly dried.

ADDITIONAL COMMENTS

Additional build-ups, of suitable material, can be added to the buttress of the pad with rubber cement and liquid latex; if additional traction is required, similar build-ups can be adhered to the dorsum of the device. The bands of elastic adhesive over the 2nd and 4th toes can be retained to ensure proper anchorage or they can be trimmed, for patient comfort or if not needed for stabilization. The appliance should be worn day and night for 4 weeks post-surgically, then removed at night.

REMOVABLE TRACTION APPLIANCE FOR FOURTH TOE

INDICATIONS
To help realign fourth toe following tenotomy surgery; to help realign a dorsally contracted fourth toe.

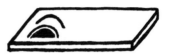

Figure 1.

MATERIALS
$\frac{1}{16}''$ Polokoff felt, $\frac{1}{2}''$ or $\frac{3}{4}''$ wide elastic adhesive, liquid latex, paper toweling, scissors.

BOUNDARIES
The appliance is worn over the 2nd, 3rd, and 4th toes with a prop in the sulcus under the same digits.

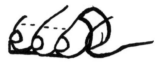

Figure 2.

CONSTRUCTION
1. Cut a $\frac{1}{16}''$ felt rectangle $3'' \times 1\frac{1}{8}''$.
2. Fold one end over $\frac{3}{4}''$.
3. Make two parallel cuts in the folded edge, $\frac{1}{2}''$ long, $\frac{3}{8}''$ in from each edge; the ring resulting is $\frac{3}{8}''$ wide and $1''$ long (Fig. 1).
4. Slip the ring over the 4th toe and fold the remaining felt along its long axis into the sulcus area beneath the middle three digits.
5. Trim the excess felt around the ring flush against the lateral border of the 4th toe; trim any excess felt extending beyond the 1st interspace (Fig. 2).
6. Remove the pad from the foot and unfold it.

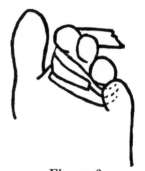

Figure 3.

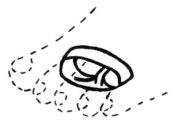

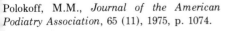

Polokoff, M.M., *Journal of the American Podiatry Association*, 65 (11), 1975, p. 1074.

Figure 4.

7. Apply liquid latex to all surfaces of the felt and blot any excess liquid by pressing the pad between sheets of paper toweling.
8. Replace the ring over the 4th toe as in Step 4 above.
9. Adhere one end of ½" or ¾" wide elastic adhesive to the fold in the felt under the 4th toe; adhere the strip to the entire length of the felt under the 3rd and 2nd toes (the felt should be nearly flattened in the area under the 2nd digit), up through the 1st interspace, over the dorsums of the 2nd, 3rd, and 4th toes, down through the 4th interspace, and back to the starting point (Fig. 3).

10. Repeat Step 9 above, so that the entire device and middle three digits have been encircled twice; continue the adhesive strip once additionally along the sulcus portion of the device, ending just at the medial aspect of the 2nd toe (Fig. 4).
11. Apply liquid latex to all surfaces of the elastic adhesive and to the felt; the appliance should be stiff when properly dried.

ADDITIONAL COMMENTS

Care must be exercised by the patient when replacing the device on the foot so that the bands do not twist.

DORSAL TENDON PAD

INDICATIONS

To help protect the tendon of extensor hallucis longus and/or a lesion over the tendon from insult.

MATERIALS

⅛" or ¼" adhesive felt, binding material, scissors.

BOUNDARIES

The pad lies over the tendon of extensor hallucis longus as it crosses the 1st metatarsophalangeal joint on the dorsum of the foot.

CONSTRUCTION

1. Cut a 1½" to 2" square of adhesive felt.
2. Skive all edges to a feather edge.
3. Fashion a groove on the adhesive surface of the pad (that surface which is to contact the skin) to accommodate the tendon; the groove should be deep enough to allow free movement of the tendon through all ranges of motion and extend from one edge of the pad to the opposite edge through the middle of the pad (Fig. 1).
4. Fashion a central cavity along

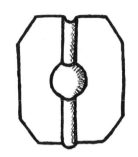

Figure 1.

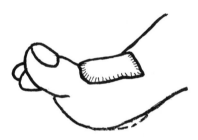

Figure 2.

the course of the groove to accommodate any lesion that may be present (optional if no lesion is present).
5. Trim the four corners of the square.
6. Adhere the pad in position over the tendon and/or lesion (Fig. 2).
7. Bind pad with an appropriate material.

Charlesworth, F., *Chiropody—Theory and Practice*, 5th Edition, London, The Actinic Press, 1961.

REMOVABLE LATEX FIFTH TOE HELOMA DURUM SHIELD MADE WITH TUBULAR GAUZE

INDICATIONS
To help relieve the symptoms of heloma durum affecting the fifth toe.

MATERIALS
¹⁄₁₆″ or ⅛″ felt, No. 1 Surgitube, rubber cement, liquid latex, hot air dryer, powder, scissors, plastic wrap or waxed paper.

BOUNDARIES
The shield is worn over the entire fifth toe.

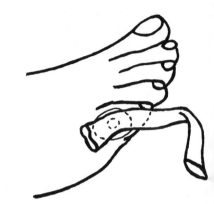

Figure 1.

CONSTRUCTION
1. Fashion an aperture pad of felt that will accommodate the lesion.
2. Adhere the aperture pad in place around the lesion with rubber cement.
3. Paint rubber cement over the surface of the felt pad and onto the entire skin surface that the completed shield will cover, i.e., the whole 5th toe and surrounding skin on dorsal, lateral, and plantar aspects.
4. Cut a 4-inch length of No. 1 Surgitube; make a 2-inch long slit up the seam of the gauze from one end.
5. Lay the uncut end of the Surgi-

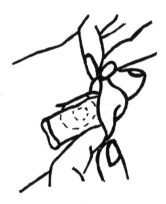

Figure 2.

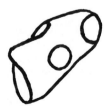

Figure 3.

Polokoff, M.M., *Journal of the American Podiatry Association*, 48 (9), 1958, p. 432.

tube over the felt shield and onto the skin just proximal to it; the gauze should adhere to the now dried rubber cement surfaces (Fig. 1).

6. Involute the cut end of the Surgitube and work the material back over the entire fifth toe, adhering it to the dried rubber cement surfaces; make certain to avoid wrinkling the gauze, especially near the nail borders (Fig. 2).

7. Adhere any loose edges of gauze to the skin with rubber cement.

8. Apply one layer of liquid latex to the entire shield; hasten drying with the hot air dryer.

9. Apply a second layer of latex; dry with hot air dryer.

10. Powder the shield on the foot and cover it with plastic wrap or waxed paper.

11. Instruct patient to wear shield for 4 to 7 days until next visit.

12. At subsequent visit, remove shield from foot and trim as necessary; cut out central hole of aperture and distal end of shield that covers nail (Fig. 3).

ADDITIONAL COMMENTS

Shield should always be powdered before patient wears it.

REMOVABLE DEVICE FOR FIFTH METATARSAL HEAD LESIONS

INDICATIONS

To help relieve the symptoms of Tailor's bunion with or without associated plantar lesions about the fifth metatarsal head.

MATERIALS

⅛" felt, alcohol, ½" wide Elastoplast, rubber cement, liquid latex, powder, hot air dryer, plastic wrap or paper toweling, scissors.

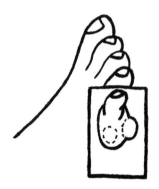

Figure 1.

BOUNDARIES

The device is worn over the 5th digit extending over the lateral aspect of the 5th ray proximal to the head of the 5th metatarsal.

CONSTRUCTION

1. Outline the lateral periphery of the 5th metatarsophalangeal joint with transferable ink (ballpoint pen).
2. Cut a rectangle, 2" × 3", from ⅛" felt.
3. Fold the rectangle in half along its long axis; cut out a semi-oval, 1¼" long and 5/16" wide, that will result in an oval ⅝" wide by 1¼" long; start the cut ¾" from one edge, so that the resultant oval is off-centered toward the distal edge.
4. Outline the plantar aspect of

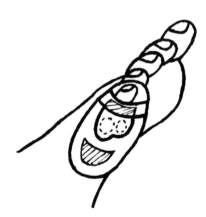

Figure 2.

   the 5th metatarsal head with transferable ink.

5. Place the pad on the foot with the distal (¾" edge) introduced into the 4th interspace

Polokoff, M.M., *Journal of the American Podiatry Association*, 57 (12), 1967, p. 556.

and the 5th digit projecting from the oval (Fig. 1).

6. Moisten the surface of the pad that lies against the skin with alcohol and press it to the skin to effect the transfer of the ink outlines.

7. Remove the pad from the foot and cut along all ink transfer lines; trim the corners of the rectangle to produce an oval-shaped pad; bevel the periphery of the felt oval.

8. Encircle the foot with a ½" wide strip of Elastoplast, non-adhesive side contacting the skin, beginning near the shaft of the 5th proximal phalanx, continuing around the foot, and then back to the starting point, adhering the two ends together somewhere on the plantar aspect of the foot.

9. Adhere the felt oval to the foot so that the bones of the Tailor's bunion, the plantar aspect of the 5th metatarsal head, and the ½" wide strip of Elastoplast are visible through the aperture that has been cut from the felt.

10. Adhere a second ½" wide strip of Elastoplast to the one encircling the foot so that the distal portion of the felt oval is "sandwiched" between the two layers of adhesive; this second Elastoplast strip need not encircle the foot, just serve to secure the felt pad to the first Elastoplast strip.

11. Apply a thin layer of liquid latex to the felt pad and to the Elastoplast strips that cover the pad; do not apply latex to the felt that lies in the 4th interspace; hasten drying with the hot air dryer.

12. Trim the Elastoplast strips that extend away from the body of the felt oval.

13. Powder the device on the foot, cover with plastic wrap or paper toweling, and replace hose and shoe.

14. Instruct patient to wear device for a minimum of 24 hours and return for adjustments.

15. At the subsequent visit, remove device and trim as necessary for patient comfort; trim away any portion of the Elastoplast strip that may impinge upon any bony prominence (Fig. 2).

ADDITIONAL COMMENTS

Appropriate build-ups should be added both proximally and distally to the lesions until they are resolved.

REMOVABLE POLYURETHANE APPLIANCES
(1—Underlapping 5th Toe; 2—Basic Apertured Crest; 3—Hallux Shield; 4—Quintus Shield; 5—Sling Crest; 6— Hallux Shield Sling; 7—Quintus Shield Sling; 8—Crest Sling; 9—Hallux Sling Shield; 10—Quintus Sling Shield)

INDICATIONS

To help relieve symptoms associated with:

1. Underlapping 5th digit.
2. Hammer digit syndrome of middle three lesser toes.
3. Hallux malleus, hallux rigidus, hallux "pinch" callus.
4. Heloma durum of 5th digit.
5. Plantar tylomata sub 2nd, 3rd, or 4th metatarsal heads, with secondary digital conditions.
6. Hallux conditions in combination with "bunion" or sesamoid conditions.
7. 5th digit conditions in combination with "Tailor's bunion" or plantar lateral 5th metatarsal head lesion.
8. Hammer digit syndrome, with secondary plantar metatarsal conditions.
9. "Bunion" or sesamoid condition.
10. "Tailor's bunion" or plantar lateral 5th metatarsal head lesion.

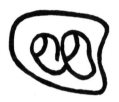

Figure 1.

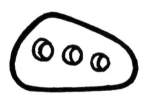

Figure 2.

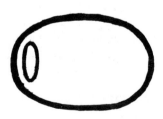

Figure 3.

Whitney, A.K., *Current Podiatry*, 13 (12), 1964, p. 20.

Fisher, C., and Whitney, A.K., Orthodigital Correction, Chapter 12 in Weinstein, F., *Principles and Practice of Podiatry*, Philadelphia, Lea & Febiger, 1968.

MATERIALS

1″ or 2″ thick medium density polyurethane foam, urethane punches, long skiving knife, prenyl punching card, scissors (these items constitute the urethane designing tray); Vultex 3E6M, pint-size plastic bags, plastic backed absorbent paper toweling, disposable plastic gloves, 1″ wide adhesive tape (these items constitute the urethan molding tray).

BOUNDARIES

The appliances are worn:
1. Over the 4th and 5th digits (Fig. 1).
2. Over the three middle toes (Fig. 2).
3. Over the entire hallux (Fig. 3).
4. Over the entire 5th toe (Fig. 4).
5. Over the three middle digits with a plantar extension to accommodate the plantar lesions (Fig. 5).
6. Over the entire hallux with a long extension to accommodate a "bunion" deformity or sesamoid lesion (Fig. 6).
7. Over the entire 5th digit with a long extension to accommodate a "Tailor's bunion" deformity or plantar lateral 5th metatarsal head lesion (Fig. 7).
8. Same as (5) above (Fig. 8).
9. Same as (6) above (Fig. 9).
10. Same as (7) above (Fig. 10).

CONSTRUCTION

1. Select the suitable urethane foam block.
2. Shape the foam block initially with the long skiving knife to the basic shape desired.

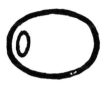

Figure 4.

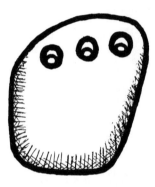

Figure 5.

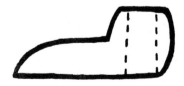

Figure 6.

3. Punch any apertures as required on the prenyl card so as not to mar any furniture surface.

4. Shape the foam with scissors to complete the desire urethane design.

5. Place the designed urethane foam in a plastic bag.

6. Add Vultex solution and squeeze the liquid into the foam until saturated.

7. Put on disposable plastic gloves.

8. Remove wet foam from bag and towel-blot excess Vultex liquid.

9. Work wet foam onto the desired digits.

10. Trim any excess foam with scissors.

11. Cover the forefoot with two plastic bags and bind bags to foot with tape.

12. Express air from bags and assist patient with replacing hose and shoes.

13. Instruct patient to leave device and bags on foot for at least five hours; after this, device can be removed and allowed to air dry; powder device well before replacing it on foot.

14. Reappoint patient within the first week.

15. At subsequent visit, examine device and trim as necessary for comfort and efficiency.

16. Repeat Steps 5 through 14 above.

17. Examine and adjust or repair device as necessary at all future visits.

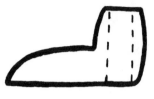

Figure 7.

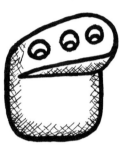

Figure 8.

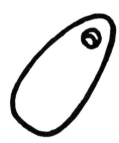

Figure 9.

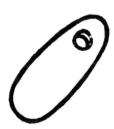

Figure 10.

Specific Sizes of Polyurethane Blocks Required for Each Appliance:

Fig. 1—2″ wide by 2″ high by 1″ deep.

Fig. 2—3″ wide by 2″ high by 2″ deep.

Fig. 3—2″ wide by 2″ high by 3″ deep.

Fig. 4—1½″ wide by 1½″ high by 2″ deep.

Fig. 5—3″ wide by 1″ high by 4″ deep.

Fig. 6—2″ wide by 2″ high by 5″ deep.

Fig. 7—1½″ wide by 2″ high by 4″ deep.

Fig. 8—3″ wide by 2″ high by 4″ deep.

Fig. 9—2″ wide by 1″ high by 5″ deep.

Fig. 10—1½″ wide by 1″ high by 4″ deep.

ADDITIONAL COMMENTS

Vultex 3E6M can be obtained from podiatry supply firms or from General Latex & Chemical Corporation, 666 Main St., Cambridge, MA.

BUTTERFLY STRAPPING FOR NAIL INVERSION

INDICATIONS
To help relieve the symptoms of onychocryptosis of the hallux; to help "train," or reduce the tendency to, nail inversion ("ingrowing").

MATERIALS
⅛" adhesive felt or adhesive moleskin, scissors.

BOUNDARIES
The strapping envelopes the hallux distally.

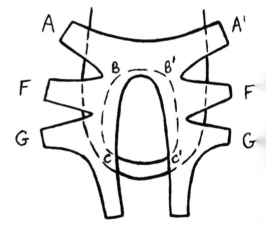

CONSTRUCTION
1. Cut a 1½" square of ⅛" felt or moleskin.
2. Trim the square to the "butterfly" configuration and make cuts shown.
3. Apply the strapping to the nail folds of the affected hallux as follows; material should not be adhered to the nail plate:

   a. Adhere flaps A and A' to the medial and lateral aspects of the skin of proximal phalanx of the hallux.

   b. Crease the edges of the material well down into the nail fold BC and B'C'; exert slight tension at D and E while doing so.

c. Pull flap D under toe toward E with tension and adhere it to skin plantar to hallux.

d. Pull flap E under toe toward D with tension and adhere it to skin plantar to hallux.

e. Pull flap F laterally with sufficient tension to evert the

Koppe, W.P., *Clinical Journal of Chiropody, Podiatry and Pedic Surgery*, 6 (5), 1934, p. 155.

nail fold tissue; adhere the flap to the skin on the side of the hallux; pull and adhere F' in the identical manner.

f. Pull flap G laterally with sufficient tension to evert the nail fold tissue; adhere the flap to the skin on the side of the hallux; pull and adhere G' in the identical manner.

VII

HEEL

Felt Heel Bar
Felt Posterior Heel Pad
Removable Posterior Heel Appliance
Strapping for Calcaneal Exostosis and Osteoma
Sponge Rubber Heel Pad
Bow-String Strapping for Painful Heel
Replaceable Heel Cup
Whale Pad
Heel Lift
Horse-Shoe Pad

FELT HEEL BAR

INDICATIONS

To help relieve the symptoms of heel fibrositis or calcaneal spur.

MATERIALS

5/16″ felt, rubber cement, scissors.

BOUNDARIES

The felt bar is worn in the shoe.

CONSTRUCTION

1. Cut a strip of felt 1½″ wide and 1″ longer than the width of the heel of the shoe.
2. Bevel the edges of the felt for patient comfort.
3. Adhere the felt into the shoe so that it spans the width of the heel just anterior to the calcaneal tuberosities; the strip should extend up onto the inner medial and lateral borders of the shoe.

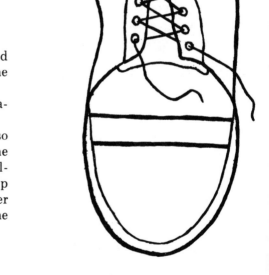

ADDITIONAL COMMENTS

The bar tends to tilt the heel posteriorly and relieves pain on the plantar surface of the foot.

Gibbard, L.C., *British Journal of Chiropody*, 23 (8), 1958, p. 203.

FELT POSTERIOR HEEL PAD

INDICATIONS
To help relieve the symptoms of posterior calcaneal bursitis.

MATERIALS
¼" adhesive felt, Elastoplast, scissors.

BOUNDARIES
The pad completely covers the posterior aspect of the heel.

CONSTRUCTION
1. Cut an egg-shaped pad from ¼" adhesive felt; skive all edges well.
2. Fashion an oval depression in the adhesive side of the pad to accommodate the painful area; the depth should be about three-quarters of the thickness of the felt.
3. Adhere the pad to the appropriate area of the heel, with the narrow end of the pad directed superiorly (Fig. 1).
4. Cut a strip of Elastoplast 2" wide by about 6" long; round the corners of the strip.
5. Adhere one end of the Elastoplast strip to the skin just beyond the superior margin of the felt pad; continue to adhere the Elastoplast to the felt pad itself and, working distally, adhere

Gibbard, L.C., *British Journal of Chiropody*, 23 (8), 1958, p. 203.

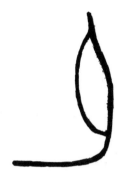

Figure 1.

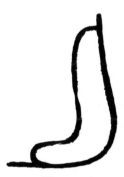

Figure 2.

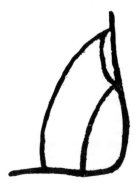

Figure 3.

the strip to the skin on the plantar aspect of the heel; the felt pad should be completely covered and anchored in place (Fig. 2).

6. Cut a second strip of Elastoplast, 1½" wide by 10" to 12" long; round the corners of the strip.

7. Adhere one end of this strip to the skin just beyond the superior margin of the first Elastoplast strip applied to the heel as well as to the first Elastoplast strip itself; continue to adhere the second strip such that all edges of the initial Elastoplast strip are completely covered and thereby firmly secured to the skin just adjacent to them (Fig. 3).

REMOVABLE POSTERIOR HEEL APPLIANCE

INDICATIONS

To help relieve the symptoms of posterior calcaneal bursitis, tenosynovitis or tendinitis of the tendo Achilles, blister or callus at the site of undue pressure, or Haglund's deformity.

MATERIALS

3/16" felt, Elastoplast, sheet of paper, cardboard, scissors.

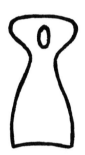

Figure 1.

BOUNDARIES

The appliance covers the entire posterior aspect of the heel and the plantar aspect of the heel.

CONSTRUCTION

1. Cut the pattern shown from a piece of paper 4" × 6" (Fig. 1).
2. Place the paper pattern on the heel; the lower portion is placed on the plantar aspect of the heel while the upper portion covers the posterior aspect of the heel; determine the painful area to be shielded and mark this area on the paper pattern.
3. Cut out an aperture that will accommodate the painful area.
4. Cut a heel insole "stiffener" from carboard that approximates the size of the lower por-

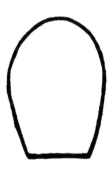

Figure 2.

tion of the paper pattern; this should be slightly smaller than the size of the heel of the shoe in which it will be worn (Fig. 2).
5. Fashion a suitable felt aperture pad from 3/16" felt that will accommodate the painful area (Fig. 3).

Koppe, W.P., *Clinical Journal of Chiropody, Podiatry and Pedic Surgery*, 5 (7), 1933, p. 229.

6. Cut two (or more) pieces of Elastoplast (or chamois) that are larger than the paper pattern, i.e., larger than 4" × 6".

7. Place the cardboard heel insole on the lower half of the adhesive surface of the Elastoplast in the approximate position determined by comparing to the paper pattern.

8. Place the felt aperture on the adhesive side of the Elastoplast in the exact position of the lesion determined by comparing to the cut-out aperture on the paper pattern.

9. Place the second piece of Elastoplast over the first, approximating the adhesive surfaces together; the cardboard heel stiffener and the felt aperture are now "sandwiched" between the two layers.

10. Place the paper pattern in position over the layered appliance, matching the positions of the aperture and heel "stiffener," and trace it onto the Elastoplast.

11. Cut out the outlined appliance; make certain all edges are firmly adhered.

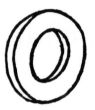

Figure 3.

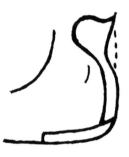

Figure 4.

12. Fit the appliance to the patient's foot, with the aperture around the painful area or lesion (Fig. 4).

13. Replace the patient's hose; this will hold the appliance in proper position on the foot.

STRAPPING FOR CALCANEAL EXOSTOSIS AND OSTEOMA

INDICATIONS
To help relieve the symptoms of calcaneal periostitis, heel spur, or atrophied heel fat pad.

MATERIALS
Elastoplast, scissors.

BOUNDARIES
The strapping envelopes the entire heel—medial, lateral, and plantar.

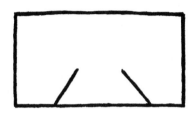

Figure 1.

CONSTRUCTION
1. Cut a rectangle of Elastoplast 4½" wide by 7" long (or as the case dictates).
2. Fold the material in half on its short axis, non-adhesive sides in contact, and make a cut approximately 2" long, at a 45 degree angle, starting about 2 inches from the open-edged border (Fig. 1).
3. Adhere one corner of the uncut edge of the plaster just inferior and anterior to the medial malleolus; adhere this edge to the skin along the medial aspect of the heel, proximal to the malleolus; pull the flap onto the plantar aspect of the heel and, being certain to pull the soft tissue structures in the same di-

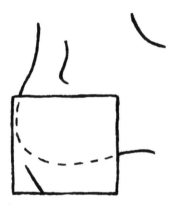

Figure 2.

rection, adhere it to the plantar surface (Fig. 2).
4. Adhere the remaining length of the uncut edge onto the posterior and lateral aspect of the heel.
5. Pull the lateral flap onto the

Koppe, W.P., *Clinical Journal of Chiropody, Podiatry and Pedic Surgery*, 5 (6), 1933, p. 184.

plantar aspect of the heel and, in the identical manner as in (3), above, adhere it to the plantar surface.

6. Pull the posterior flap onto the plantar aspect of the heel and, similarly, adhere it to the plantar surface, which should now be covered with the first two layers of Elastoplast from the medial and lateral flaps.

7. Smooth the entire strapping; avoid wrinkles.

ADDITIONAL COMMENTS

When properly applied, this strapping will "cup" all the soft tissues beneath and around the inferior aspect of the calcaneus; this can provide immediate relief to the straining plantar fascia as it pulls the periosteum at its insertion onto the calcaneus. This strapping can also be employed as the heel lock for a Campbell's Rest Strap.

SPONGE RUBBER HEEL PAD

INDICATIONS
To help relieve the symptoms of heel spur, plantar fasciitis, calcaneal periostitis.

MATERIALS
½″ sponge rubber, skiving knife, scissors.

BOUNDARIES
The pad extends over the entire plantar aspect of the calcaneus.

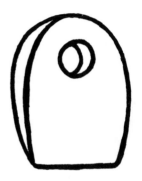

CONSTRUCTION
1. Cut a rectange of ½″ sponge rubber that is as wide as the affected heel and as long as the distance from the proximal border of the heel to about midway in the longitudinal arch.
2. Round the proximal end of the rectangle to the contour of the heel.

3. Starting from the midpoint of the length of the rectangle, skive the rubber to a featheredge distally.
4. Cut out a suitable aperture positioned at the site of the insertion of the plantar fascia to the calcaneus.
5. Place pad in heel of shoe or adhere to foot itself with suitable binding.

Healy, F., *Chiropody Record*, 17 (5), 1934, p. 119.

BOW-STRING STRAPPING FOR PAINFUL HEEL

INDICATIONS
To help relieve the symptoms of heel spur, plantar fasciitis, calcaneal periostitis.

MATERIALS
¼″ adhesive felt, 2″, 3″, and 4″ wide tape or Elastoplast, scissors.

BOUNDARIES
The strapping covers the entire plantar aspect of the foot from the metatarsal heads proximal, with several strips anchored to the upper one-third of the leg.

CONSTRUCTION
1. Cut a pad from ¼″ adhesive felt that is the size of the heel of the shoe; skive the distal half of the pad to a feather-edge.
2. Cut a suitable aperture that accommodates the painful area on the heel.
3. Adhere the felt pad to the foot with the aperture properly positioned to shield the painful area.
4. Attach one end of a 3″ or 4″ wide strip of tape to the posterior aspect of the heel (below the level of insertion of the tendo Achilles) and pull it distally to the heads of the metatarsals; adhere the distal end to

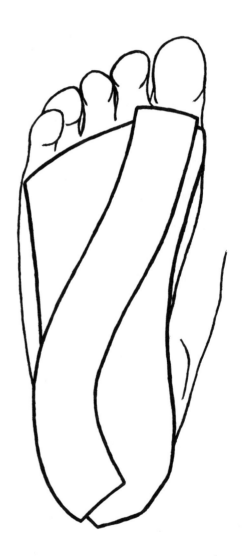

Rice, E., *Journal of the National Association of Chiropodists*, 22 (11), 1932, p. 18.

the first metatarsal head initially, then to the 2nd, 3rd, and 4th metatarsal heads; a "bow-string" is now apparent, the tape forming the string, and the plantar longitudinal arch, the bow.

5. Adhere the tape to the plantar aspect of the foot, pressing firmly, distal to proximal.
6. Adhere one end of a 2″ strip of tape to the posterior lateral surface of the heel and pull it distally to the base of the hallux; adhere the distal end here; again a "bow-string" is seen.
7. Adhere the length of this tape to the plantar surface of the foot.
8. Adhere one end of a 3″ strip of tape to the medial plantar surface of the heel; place the foot and ankle in their respective neutral positions and, while maintaining these, pass the strip of tape superiorly over the medial malleolus and adhere the other end to the inner aspect of the upper one-third of the leg; again the "bow-string" appears.
9. Adhere the length of this strip to the inner surface of the leg inferiorly to the foot.
10. Repeat (8) and (9) above for a strip of tape that is to be adhered to the lateral aspect of the leg.
11. Adhere one end of a 3″ strip of tape to the medial plantar surface of the heel; pass the strip superiorly and adhere it over the medial malleolus; con-

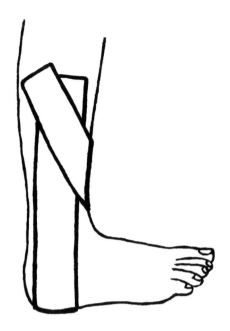

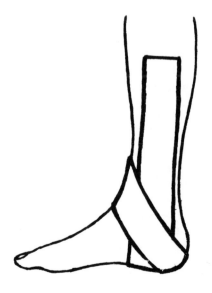

tinue adhering the strip, in a spiral fashion, to the anterior aspect of the lower one-third of the leg, and finish by adhering the other end of the strip to the lateral surface of the middle one-third of the leg.

REPLACEABLE HEEL CUP

INDICATIONS

To help relieve the symptoms of heel spur, plantar fasciitis, inferior calcaneal bursitis, calcaneal periostitis.

MATERIALS

$\frac{1}{16}''$ adhesive felt, $\frac{3}{16}''$ adhesive foam, adhesive stockinette, scissors.

BOUNDARIES

The appliance envelopes the entire heel—medial, lateral, and plantar.

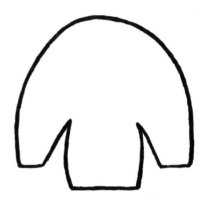

CONSTRUCTION

1. Cut a piece of $\frac{1}{16}''$ adhesive felt to the shape shown; the middle flap should be the size of the plantar aspect of the heel and the surrounding portion should be of sufficient size to envelop the heel, medially and laterally, just inferior to the malleoli.

2. Position the felt on the foot, felt surface in contact with the skin, with the middle flap on the plantar surface of the heel.

3. Fold one of the outer flaps onto the plantar aspect of the heel and adhere it to the felt there (the felt surface of the outer flap to the adhesive surface of the middle flap).

4. In a similar fashion to (3) above, fold and adhere the other outer flap to the plantar aspect of the heel.

5. Fashion a plantar heel pad from $\frac{3}{16}''$ adhesive foam the size of the affected heel; bevel all edges.

6. Adhere the foam pad to the undersurface of the felt heel cup in place on the foot (the adhesive surface of the foam to the adhesive surface of the felt).

7. If protection for a posterior heel lesion is required, cut an oval-shaped aperture pad from $\frac{3}{16}''$ adhesive foam and adhere it to the proper position on the posterior aspect of the felt heel cup in place on the foot.

8. Cover the entire exterior sur-

Dowdeswell-Childs, T.G., *The Chiropodist*, 21 (1), 1966, p. 4.

face of the heel cup, with the attached plantar heel and posterior heel pads, with adhesive stockinette.

9. Trim as necessary.

ADDITIONAL COMMENTS

If adhesive stockinette is not available, spray the entire exterior surface of the heel cup with adhesive and cover it with regular, non-adhesive, stockinette.

WHALE PAD

INDICATIONS

To remove pressure from a painful heel while supporting the long arch to limit pronation.

MATERIALS

¼" adhesive felt, skiving knife, adhesive tape.

BOUNDARIES

The boundaries are the same as those indicated for the Mayo Pad. However, an extension is incorporated that begins at the talonavicular articulation and narrows to follow the posterior border of the heel. The width tapers laterally then continues around to the aspect of the heel terminating proximal to the weight-bearing medial tuberosity of the calcaneus.

CONSTRUCTION

1. Cut the ¼" adhesive felt into a shape approximating a 4" × 8" rectangle.
2. Lightly adhere the felt to the plantar aspect of the foot. The length of the pad extends from just proximal to the metatarsal heads to the posterior aspect of the heel. The lateral border should extend to the fourth interspace and the medial border extends superiorly to meet

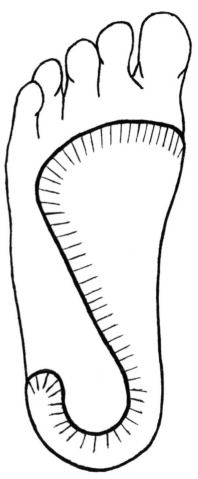

Figure 1.

the talonavicular articulation on the medial side of the foot.
3. With a pencil outline the pad as shown using the borders as indicated for the Mayo Pad but with the heel extension added as shown in Figure 1.

4. Remove the pad from the foot and cut the pad until the shape approximates the shape of a whale.

5. Skive the long arch area of the pad the same as directed for the Mayo Pad. The heel loop or "tail" area is skived abruptly on all edges making sure to leave as much flat surface as possible for the heel to rest on.

6. Adhere the pad to the foot so that the long arch area is sup- ported from the first metatarsal head to the talonavicular articulation. The heel loop should follow the posterior border of the heel without terminating directly beneath the weight-bearing tuberosity of the heel.

ADDITIONAL COMMENTS

Wherever necessary, the pad can be anchored to the foot with strips of adhesive tape to provide longer wearing time.

HEEL LIFT

INDICATIONS

Gastrocnemius, soleus, gastrocnemius/soleus, hamstring, or iliopsoas equinus; Achilles tendonitis, limb length discrepancy syndrome, shin splints, Sever's disease, retrocalcaneal bursitis.

RELATIVE CONTRAINDICATIONS

Lateral ankle sprain and/or instability; forefoot/metatarsal capsulitis or bursitis; later stages of pregnancy.

MATERIALS

Many types of materials may be employed to fabricate a heel raise; felt is customarily used, but because of its compressibility, it is no longer the material of choice; the material chosen should not "bottom out" or compress on weightbearing or after prolonged use; recommended materials include kores, laminates of leather, neoprene, and others.

BOUNDARIES

The heel lift should cover the entire plantar aspect of the rearfoot and midfoot and should be skived anteriorly to the metatarsal heads.

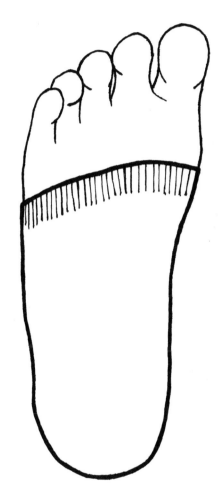

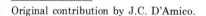

Original contribution by J.C. D'Amico.

CONSTRUCTION

1. Trace the insole from the patient's shoe; mark the positions of the first and fifth metatarsal heads.
2. Cut out this form and duplicate it on the material desired.

3. Skive the anterior edge of the material ending just proximal to the metatarsal heads.
4. Place the material into the patient's shoe.

ADDITIONAL COMMENTS
By elevating the calcaneus, thereby plantarflexing the foot on the leg, a new increased joint range of motion is established. The tension on the posterior group muscles, such as gastrocnemius/soleus and the hamstrings, is reduced.

HORSE-SHOE PAD

INDICATIONS
To help relieve the symptoms of heel spur syndrome, plantar fasciitis, or other painful plantar heel conditions.

MATERIALS
¼" or ½" adhesive felt, adhesive foam, or sponge rubber, scissors, skiving knife.

BOUNDARIES
The pad is placed onto the plantar aspect of the heel so that it covers the medial, lateral, and posterior edges, while the central area of the heel remains exposed.

CONSTRUCTION
1. Cut a pad from ¼" or ½" thick adhesive felt, adhesive foam, or sponge rubber that is the size of the entire plantar aspect of the heel.
2. Skive the pad from about the middle of its length to a feather edge distally.
3. Cut the pad into a horse-shoe shape by trimming the central portion of the material away; leave a ½" to ¾" wide border to cover the medial, lateral, and posterior edges; round distal edges.

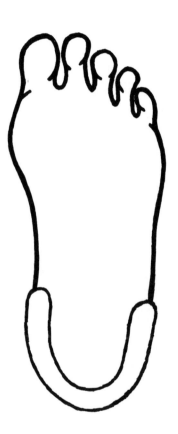

4. Adhere the pad in place onto the plantar aspect of the heel; if desired, the pad may be adhered to the interior aspect of the heel of the shoe.

VIII

STRAPPINGS

Short Tibial Strapping
Gibney Ankle Strap
  (Basketweave)
J-Strap
Reverse "J"
Cross Over J-Strap
Heel Lock
Plantar Rest Strap
  (Campbell's)
Low-Dye Strap
High-Dye Strapping
Plantar Figure of Eight
Plantar Figure of Eight with
  Separate Strips

Ankle Figure of Eight
Spica Toe Dressing
Campbell's Posterior Rest
  Strap
Flabby Heel Dressing (Heel
  Cup)
Three Layered Arch Support
Louisiana Heel Lock
Achilles Tendon Strap
Traction Sling for
  Underlapping Fifth Toe
Traction Sling for Overlapping
  Fifth Toe

SHORT TIBIAL STRAPPING

INDICATIONS

To alleviate the pain of a heel spur and other symptoms associated with a pull on the plantar fascia and long plantar ligament.

MATERIALS

2″ adhesive tape approximately 15″ long and 2 pieces of 1″ adhesive tape 2″ long.

BOUNDARIES

Extends from the dorsum of the 5th metatarsal along the plantar aspect to the anterior one-third of the tibia.

CONSTRUCTION

1. Cut a piece of 2″ adhesive tape approximately 15″ long. Apply skin adherent to the affected areas.
2. Place one end over the dorsum of the 5th metatarsal and bring the strip along the plantar aspect.
3. After coming over the medial aspect run the remainder of the tape diagonally so it extends up the anterior of the tibia.
4. Apply moderately firm tension as you apply the tape. Secure both free edges with anchor strips.

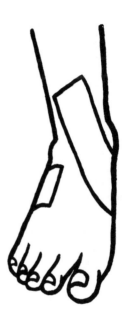

ADDITIONAL COMMENTS

1. The author also recommends higher heeled shoes, a longitudinal arch pad and the possible use of a balanced orthosis to relieve symptoms.
2. If there is a pulling on the lower tibia, the top of the strapping is loosened and foot plantarflexed. Then press the tape against the skin.

GIBNEY ANKLE STRAP (BASKETWEAVE)

INDICATIONS

To prevent inversion and eversion of the ankle to occur while allowing plantarflexion and dorsiflexion. Usage is primarily for ligamentous sprains and tendon injuries to prevent motion. This strapping is also very common before athletic competition to stabilize the ankle.

MATERIALS

1" adhesive tape cut into strips. The size of each strip and the number needed is dependent on the size of the ankle.

BOUNDARIES

Runs on the medial and lateral side of the leg 5" above the malleoli. It extends from the medial and lateral side of the foot just proximal to the first and fifth metatarsal heads.

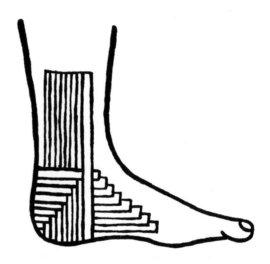

CONSTRUCTION

1. Hold the ankle in its neutral position with the foot 90° to the leg or slightly plantarflexed.
2. Place the first piece of tape 5" above the medial malleolus on the medial aspect of the leg near the Achilles tendon. Bring the strip under the heel and on the lateral side of the leg to 5" above the lateral malleolus.
3. The second strip starts proximal to the 1st metatarsal head around the medial border of the foot, across the heel and extends just proximal to the head of the 5th metatarsal.
4. The next strip runs perpendicular and overlaps the first strip by ½" and runs parallel to this strip.
5. The fourth strip runs horizontal and overlaps the second strip by ½" and runs parallel to this strip.
6. Continue this pattern until the basketweave effect is achieved.

J-STRAP

INDICATION
To prevent eversion of the calcaneus. Used primarily for medial
ligamentous injury following eversion sprains.

MATERIALS
1½" or 2" adhesive strip.

BOUNDARIES
Extends from the lateral side of the
foot just inferior to the lateral
malleolus to the middle of the
medial aspect of the leg.

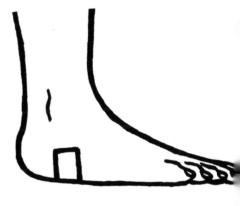

Figure 1.

CONSTRUCTION
1. Measure and cut a piece of tape
   to cover the boundaries indicated.
2. Place one end of the strip just inferior to the lateral malleolus on
   the lateral side of the foot (Fig.
   1).
3. Exert pressure as the strap
   comes under the heel and onto
   the medial side of the leg about
   half-way up (Fig. 2).

ADDITIONAL COMMENTS
1" adhesive tape anchors can be put
over the ends of the strap to secure
it in place.

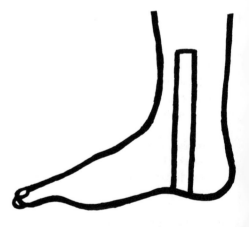

Figure 2.

REVERSE "J"

INDICATIONS

To accomplish the opposite of the J-strap by limiting inversion of the calcaneus. Used primarily for lateral ligamentous injury following inversion sprains.

MATERIALS

1½" or 2" adhesive tape strip.

BOUNDARIES

Extends from the medial side of the foot just inferior to the medial malleolus to the middle of the lateral side of the leg.

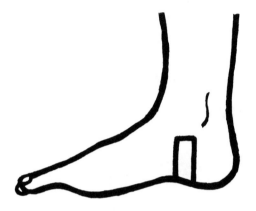

Figure 1.

CONSTRUCTION

1. Measure and cut a piece of tape to cover the boundaries indicated.
2. Place one end of the strip just inferior to the medial malleolus on the medial aspect of the heel (Fig. 1).
3. Apply tension as the tape is put under the heel and upwards on the lateral aspect of the leg about half-way up (Fig. 2).

ADDITIONAL COMMENTS

1" adhesive tape anchors can be put over the ends of the strap to secure it in place.

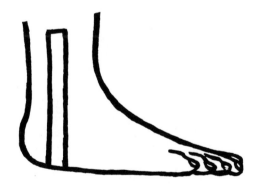

Figure 2.

CROSS OVER J-STRAP

INDICATIONS

To stop pronation by preventing adduction and plantarflexion of the talus. It also takes the strain off the anterior tibial tendon.

MATERIALS

2 or 3 strips of 2″ adhesive tape.

BOUNDARIES

Extends on the lateral aspect of the foot posterior to the base of the 5th metatarsal then under the arch and onto the anterior lateral aspect of the leg two-thirds of the way up.

CONSTRUCTION

1. Measure and cut 2 or 3 pieces of tape to cover the boundaries indicated.
2. Apply one strip just posterior to the 5th metatarsal base on the lateral aspect of the foot (Fig. 1).
3. Extend this strip with tension across the medial arch over the talo-navicular joint.
4. This strip ends on the anterior lateral two-thirds of the leg as it crossed in front of the medial malleolus (Fig. 2).
5. Apply a second or third piece of tape for additional support covering the same boundaries.

ADDITIONAL COMMENTS

1″ adhesive tape anchors can be put over the ends of the strap to secure it in place.

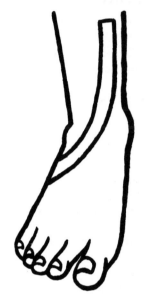

Figure 1.

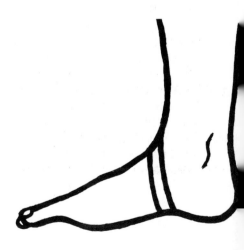

Figure 2.

HEEL LOCK

INDICATIONS

To be used for plantar fasciitis and associated heel spur syndrome. It also relieves pressure over the talo-navicular joint.

MATERIALS

One strip of 1″ adhesive tape.

BOUNDARIES

Extends from the lateral aspect just proximal to the 5th metatarsal head to the medial aspect just distal to the first metatarsal head.

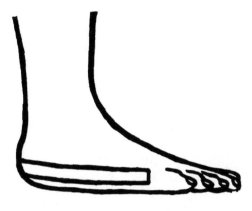

Figure 1.

CONSTRUCTION

1. Measure and cut one strip of 1″ adhesive tape to fit the above boundaries.
2. Place one end on the lateral aspect of the foot just proximal to the 5th metatarsal head (Fig. 1).
3. Place the tape around the foot onto the medial side. The strip should end just distal to the 1st metatarsal head (Fig. 2).

ADDITIONAL COMMENTS

1. Usually used in conjunction with a Plantar Rest Strap.
2. Also used frequently with a longitudinal pad for the indications above.

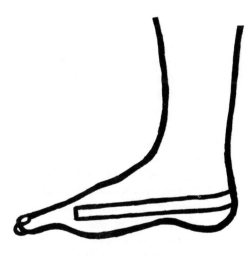

Figure 2.

PLANTAR REST STRAP (CAMPBELL'S)

INDICATIONS
To reduce strain and pressure on the plantar on the foot including the plantar fascia.

MATERIALS
3-4 strips of 1½" or 2" adhesive tape and 2 anchor strips of 1" adhesive tape.

BOUNDARIES
Runs from the lateral to medial sides of the foot covering the plantar aspect just beneath the malleoli.

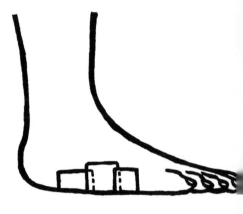

Figure 1.

CONSTRUCTION
1. Measure and cut 4 strips of 1½" or 2" adhesive tape to the desired length.
2. Apply the first strip on the lateral aspect of the foot just below the malleoli. Cross the plantar surface and attach the strip on the medial aspect to the top of the navicular (Figs. 1, 2).
3. The second strip is put on distal to the first and overlapping by one-third. It runs parallel to the first and maintains the same boundaries.
4. The third and fourth pieces are also put on distally and overlapping the preceding strip by one-third.
5. The strapping is finished with 2 horizontal anchors of 1" tape (Fig. 3).

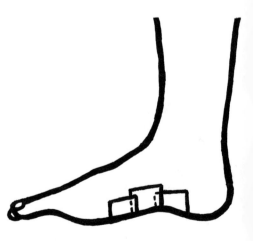

Figure 2.

ADDITIONAL COMMENTS

1. Usually used in conjunction with a longitudinal arch pad or other plantar padding.
2. A heel lock can be applied with this strapping to form a Low-Dye Strap.
3. Be especially careful not to wrinkle the skin while applying the tape.
4. Modifications to give additional support can be made. These modifications are then covered with the rest strap as described above. The modifications are:

    a. A two-inch strip is placed from the center of the heel posterior to the substentaculum tali and extends to the posterior of the metatarsal heads.

    b. Two one-inch strips run from the center of the heel to: (1) posterior of the 1st metatarsal head, and (2) posterior of the 5th metatarsal head.

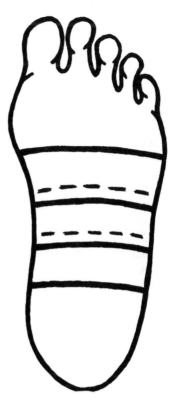

Figure 3.

LOW-DYE STRAP

INDICATIONS
To alleviate the strain associated with pronation. Primarily used for plantar fasciitis, heel spur syndrome and other symptoms caused by pronation at the mid-tarsal joint.

MATERIALS
One strip of 1″ adhesive tape, four strips of 1½″ or 2″ adhesive tape and two strips of 1″ adhesive tape anchors.

BOUNDARIES
Same boundaries as indicated in the Heel Lock and the Plantar Rest Strap.

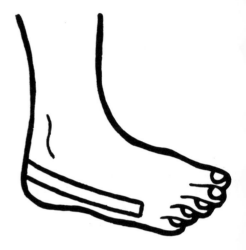

Figure 1.

CONSTRUCTION
1. Apply a Heel Lock as previously described. Before securing the tape on the medial aspect, adduct the forefoot slightly. This will hold the hallux towards the mid-line of the body (Fig. 1).
2. Over the Heel Lock apply a Plantar Rest Strap as previously applied including the horizontal anchors (Fig. 2).

ADDITIONAL COMMENTS
1. Paddings are usually used in conjunction with this strapping (e.g., Longitudinal Arch pad).
2. Bearing weight on the affected foot without wearing shoegear has a tendency to loosen this strapping.

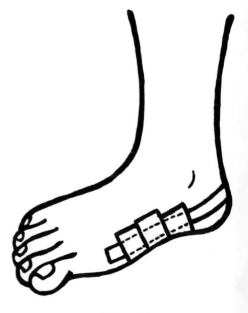

Figure 2.

HIGH-DYE STRAPPING

INDICATIONS
To be used for same indications as the Low-Dye Strapping but with greater symptoms from excessive pronation.

MATERIALS
The same materials needed to make a Low-Dye Strapping and the Cross Over J-Strap.

BOUNDARIES
The same boundaries as the Low-Dye Strap and the Cross Over J-Strap.

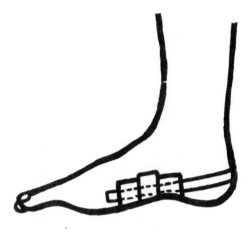

Figure 2.

CONSTRUCTION
1. Apply the Low-Dye Strap as previously described (Figs. 1, 2).
2. Now apply the Cross Over J-Strap over the Low-Dye Strap (Fig. 3).

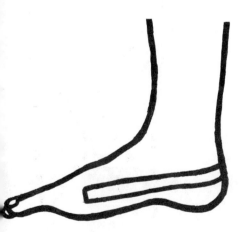

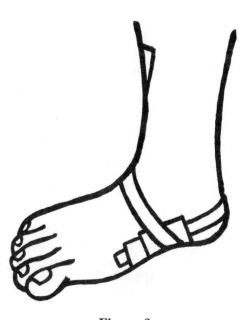

Figure 1.

Figure 3.

PLANTAR FIGURE OF EIGHT

INDICATIONS
To alleviate plantar fasciitis, heel pain and give support to the longitudinal arch.

MATERIALS
One strip of 2″ adhesive tape.

BOUNDARIES
From the posterior aspect of the calcaneus just below the insertion of the Achilles tendon one strip proceeds like a Heel Lock while the other strips cross the plantar of the foot obliquely securing just behind the heads of the 1st and 5th metatarsals on the dorsum of the foot.

CONSTRUCTION
1. Measure and cut a strip of 2″ tape to reach behind the heads of the 1st and 5th metatarsals.
2. Cut the tape in half from both ends leaving ½″ intact in the center of the strip.
3. Fix the intact portion to the posterior of the heel just below the tendo-Achilles insertion (Fig. 1).
4. The top 1″ strip is applied obliquely over the plantar of the foot. The lateral strip attaches just proximal to the 1st metatarsal head. The medial strip attaches just proximal to the 5th metatarsal head. This top strip

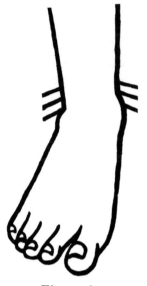

Figure 1.

Figure 2.

has created an X over the plantar of the foot (Fig. 2).

5. The bottom 1″ strip is then attached in the same manner as a Heel Lock (Fig. 3).

ADDITIONAL COMMENTS

A Plantar Rest Strap can be used over this strapping.

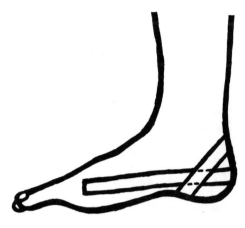

Figure 3.

PLANTAR FIGURE OF EIGHT WITH SEPARATE STRIPS

INDICATIONS
To give additional support to the longitudinal arch and alleviate the symptoms as described previously for the Plantar Figure of Eight.

MATERIALS
6 strips of 1″ adhesive tape.

BOUNDARIES
The boundaries are the same as in the Plantar Figure of Eight.

CONSTRUCTION
1. Measure and cut 6 strips as indicated.
2. Start one strip just proximal to the first metatarsal head on the medial aspect.
3. Run this strip obliquely across the plantar aspect and encircle the heel. Now, bring the strip along the medial aspect of the foot and end it by the head of the 1st metatarsal (Fig. 1).
4. The second strip starts on the lateral aspect of the foot proximal to the 5th metatarsal head.
5. Run this strip obliquely across the plantar aspect and encircle the heel. Now, bring the strip along the lateral aspect of the foot and end it by the head of the 5th metatarsal (Fig. 2).
6. Overlap each of these strips twice with the same boundaries.

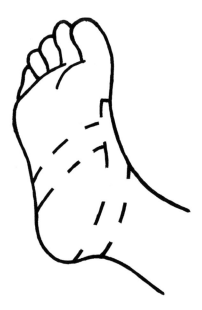

Figure 1.

ADDITIONAL COMMENTS
 A Plantar Rest Strap can be used
 over this strapping.

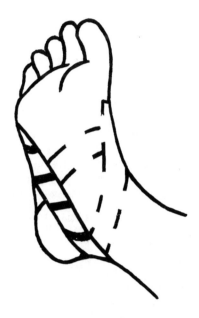

Figure 2.

ANKLE FIGURE OF EIGHT

INDICATIONS
To prevent inversion and eversion of the calcaneus while also stopping plantarflexion of the foot.

MATERIALS
4-6 strips of 1″ adhesive tape.

BOUNDARIES
Covers the entire ankle area on all aspects.

CONSTRUCTION
1. Hold the foot in the position desired.
2. Place the first strip at the upper posterior aspect of the ankle on the lateral side. Come around the lateral side above the malleoli to the medial side below the malleoli. Continue this strip across the plantar of the foot, obliquely across the anterior of the leg onto the medial side. The strip ends where it began at the upper posterior aspect of the ankle (Fig. 1).
3. The second strip overlaps the first piece by one-third and runs parallel to it on the distal aspect.
4. Continue with 4-6 strips until the ankle is covered and the proper immobilization accomplished (Fig. 2).

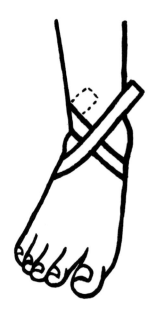

Figure 1.

ADDITIONAL COMMENTS

1. Bony prominences can be padded with webril, etc., before taping.
2. Instead of separate strips, this strapping can be applied with one continuous piece. Continue this piece until the ankle is covered and the proper immobilization achieved.

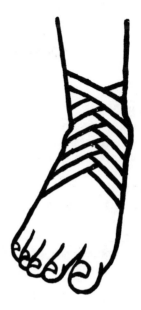

Figure 2.

SPICA TOE DRESSING

INDICATIONS
To immobilize a digit after fracture or dislocation or following postoperative surgical procedures.

MATERIALS
4-6 strips of ⅛" or ¼" adhesive tape 3"-4" long.

BOUNDARIES
Covers the entire digit on all aspects.

CONSTRUCTION
1. Start the first strip on the dorsal medial aspect of the affected toe at its base. Extend the strip obliquely to the lateral aspect of the toe, across the plantar of the toe and obliquely back to the lateral aspect on the dorsum at the base of the toe.
2. The second strip attaches just lateral to the first strip and runs parallel to that strip.
3. Continue with overlapping strips until the entire toe is encircled with tape and properly immobilized.

ADDITIONAL COMMENTS
1. Obviously the tape is applied

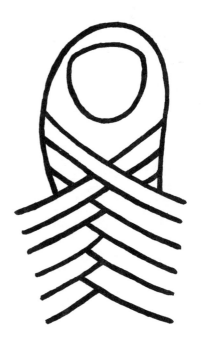

over the sterile dressing when used postoperatively.
2. It is extremely important to tape the toe in the correct position so that healing occurs in the desired position.

CAMPBELL'S POSTERIOR REST STRAP

INDICATIONS

To alleviate strain from the Achilles tendon and support the posterior muscle group of the leg; also for Achilles tendonitis, plantaris tendon rupture and calcaneal apophysitis.

MATERIALS

3 strips of 1" adhesive tape approximately 18" long and 3 strips of 2" adhesive tape 4"-6" long.

BOUNDARIES

Extends from the plantar of the Lisfranc's joint up the posterior two-thirds of the lower leg.

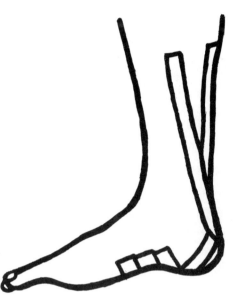

Figure 1.

CONSTRUCTION

1. Apply the first 18" strip of tape starting at the plantar medial aspect of the foot inferior to the 1st cuneiform. Extend this piece obliquely towards the lateral aspect of the heel and up the lateral side of the lower leg.

2. Apply the second 18" strip of tape starting at the plantar lateral aspect of the foot inferior to the base of the 5th metatarsal. Extend this piece obliquely toward the medial aspect of the heel and up the medial side of the lower leg (Fig. 1).

3. The third equal strip starts plantar to Lisfranc's joint in the center of the foot. Extend this strip posteriorly over the heel and up the center of the lower leg.

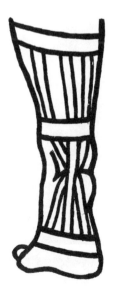

Figure 2.

4. Apply the first 2″ anchor around the leg just superior to the ankle joint. The anchor strips are applied 90° to the original strips.

5. The last two 2″ anchors are applied at the ends of the 1″ tape (Fig. 2).

ADDITIONAL COMMENTS

1. A heel lift in the shoe is also effective in conjunction with this strapping.

2. The tape should be applied with the foot mildly plantarflexed. Apply tension while applying the 1″ strips will further plantarflex the foot.

FLABBY HEEL DRESSING (HEEL CUP)

INDICATIONS
To alleviate acute heel pain, support the heel and secure excessive soft tissue around the heel.

MATERIALS
3″-4″ elastic tape, 2 strips of 2″ adhesive tape and 1 strip of 1″ adhesive tape for the anchor.

BOUNDARIES
Covers the entire plantar of the heel, extends just proximal to both malleoli and across the mid tarsal joint on the medial and lateral aspects of the foot.

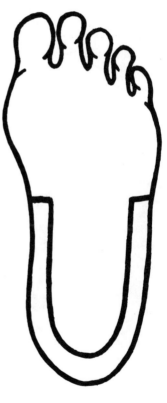

Figure 2.

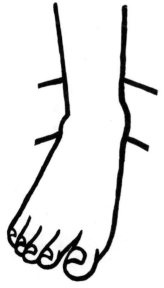

Figure 1.

CONSTRUCTION

1. Measure and cut the piece of 3"-4" elastic tape so that without tension it reaches around the posterior of the heel to reach 2 cm proximal to the mid tarsal joint on the medial and lateral sides.
2. Place this tape over the posterior of the heel so that 1" extends onto the plantar aspect. Pull the tape with tension and apply it on the sides of the foot (Fig. 1).
3. Secure the plantar edge onto the skin and avoid overlap of the tape (Fig. 2).
4. Place a strip of 2" adhesive tape over the plantarmost aspect of the heel that ends below both medial and lateral malleoli.
5. Take a second piece of 2" adhesive tape and place it proximal to the first piece with about a ½" of overlap (Fig. 3).
6. Now place a 1" strip of adhesive tape over the superior aspect of this dressing to act as the anchor (Fig. 4).

ADDITIONAL COMMENTS

If the tape should overlap, continue to flatten the strapping as much as possible. Using the heel of the scissors, cut this overlap off as flat as possible. Now the strapping should conform perfectly to the shape of the foot without any overlap or bulges.

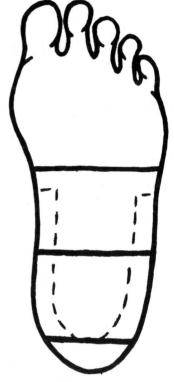

Figure 3.

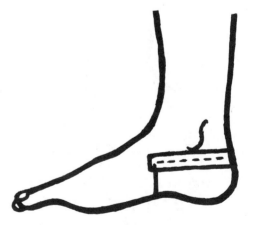

Figure 4.

THREE LAYERED ARCH SUPPORT

INDICATIONS
To prevent the symptoms of excessive pronation and support the plantar aspect of the foot.

MATERIALS
2 1" strips of adhesive tape 3" long, 1 1" strip of adhesive tape 6"-8" long, 3 1" strips of adhesive tape 8" long, the materials necessary for making 2 Plantar Rest Straps, and 1 1" strip for an anchor approximately 12" long.

BOUNDARIES
Same boundaries as indicated in the Plantar Rest Strap.

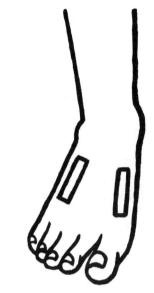

Figure 1.

CONSTRUCTION
1. Hold the foot slightly supinated while applying the tape.
2. Place the first 3" strip on the dorsal medial aspect of the foot just proximal to the 1st MPJ.
3. Place the second 3" strip on the dorsal lateral aspect of the foot just proximal to the 5th MPJ (Fig. 1).
4. Take the 6"-8" strip and place it around the heel overlapping the first two strips by 1". The tape should be inferior to the Achilles insertion (Fig. 2).
5. Apply a Plantar Rest Strap as previously described.

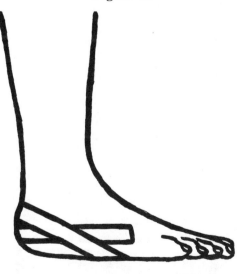

Figure 2.

6. Place the first 8″ strip of 1″ tape under the head of the 3rd metatarsal and continue posteriorly onto the back of the heel.

7. Place the second 8″ strip of 1″ tape under the 5th metatarsal head and continue obliquely onto the medial aspect of the heel.

8. Place the last 8″ strip of 1″ tape under the 1st metatarsal head and continue obliquely onto the lateral aspect of the heel (Fig. 3).

9. Apply another Plantar Rest Strap as in Step 5.

10. Use a 1″ anchor to cover all the free margins as a Heel Lock (Fig. 4).

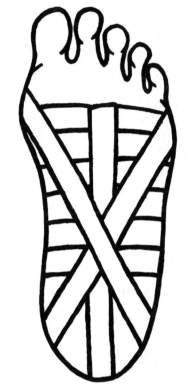

Figure 3.

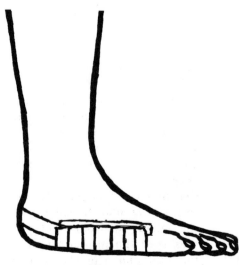

Figure 4.

LOUISIANA HEEL LOCK

INDICATIONS

To prevent the symptoms of excessive pronation, used for ankle sprains, ankle strains and shin splints.

MATERIALS

Continuous wrap of 1″ adhesive tape, 3″ × 3″ gauze or webril, and 2 1″ strips of adhesive tape for anchors.

BOUNDARIES

Covers the entire ankle on all its borders.

CONSTRUCTION

1. Protect the anterior of the ankle and both malleoli using webril or gauze.
2. Start the wrap with 1″ tape on the dorsal lateral surface of the foot (Fig. 1).
3. Roll the tape around the foot, under the arch onto the lateral side (Fig. 2).
4. Continue the wrap over the dorsum, around the ankle, across the heel below the Achilles insertion, across the lateral heel and across the plantar surface (Figs. 3, 4).
5. Continue the wrap onto the dorsum and around the ankle, over the lateral malleolus and proceed over the medial aspect of the heel and over the plantar (Figs. 5, 6).

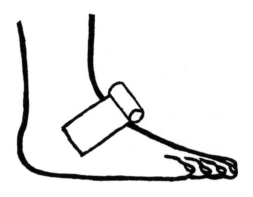

Figure 1.

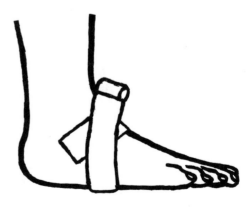

Figure 2.

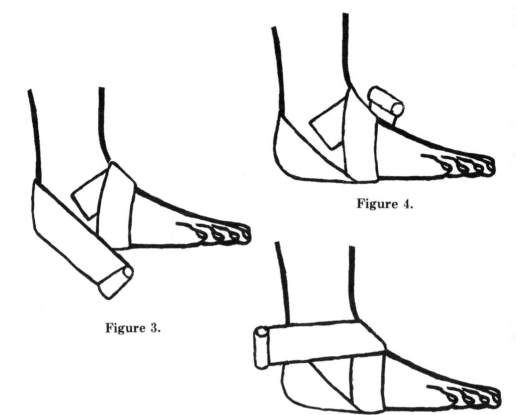

Figure 3.

Figure 4.

Figure 5.

6. The wrap now covers the dorsum, goes around the ankle covering both malleoli and ends after the medial malleolus (Figs. 7, 8).
7. Use 1″ tape as anchors over any free edges. Apply a 1″ strip around the heel to the dorsal surface of the foot as an additional lock.

ADDITIONAL COMMENTS

Be careful not to compromise the circulation by applying this wrap too tightly.

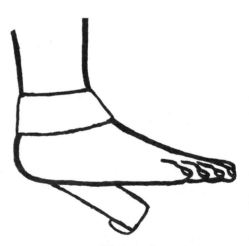

Figure 6.

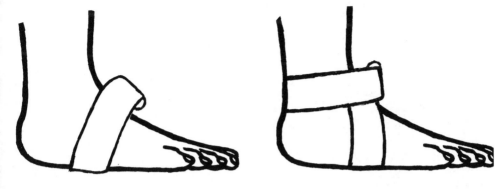

Figure 7.   Figure 8.

ACHILLES TENDON STRAP

INDICATIONS
To alleviate pressure on the Achilles tendon and used for Achilles tendon sprain or strain.

MATERIALS
2 1″ strips of adhesive tape for anchors, 3-4 1″ strips of adhesive tape 12″ long, 4 1″ strips of adhesive tape 4″ long and materials necessary for a Plantar Rest Strap.

BOUNDARIES
Extends on the plantar of the foot from the metatarsal heads to 3″-4″ above the malleoli on the posterior lower leg.

CONSTRUCTION
1. Place a 1″ anchor strip around the leg 3″-4″ above the malleoli.
2. Place a second 1″ anchor strip on the plantar surface by the metatarsal heads (Fig. 1).
3. Place 3-4 strips of 1″ tape from the metatarsal heads posteriorly over the calcaneus and on the back of the leg to meet the first anchor strip. These strips follow the course of the Achilles tendon (Fig. 2).
4. Bind the tape down at the top free edge. Bind around the ankle with 3 4″ strips to secure the tape to the ankle (Fig. 3).
5. Apply a Plantar Rest Strap as previously described.

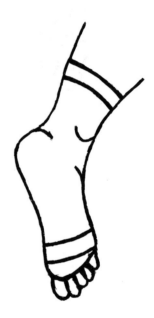

Figure 1.

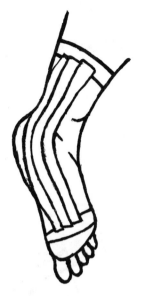

Figure 2.

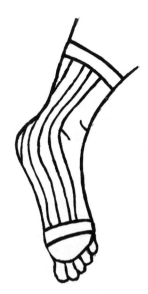

Figure 3.

TRACTION SLING FOR UNDERLAPPING FIFTH TOE

INDICATIONS
To help correct the position of an underlapping 5th toe deformity.

MATERIALS
¾″ to 1″ strip rubber, rubber cement, scissors.

BOUNDARIES
The device looped over the fifth digit, with a length of strip rubber passing obliquely across the dorsal aspect of the foot (from distal lateral to proximal medial) and around the ankle.

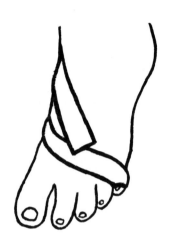

CONSTRUCTION
1. Cut a ¾″ to 1″ wide strip of rubber to an 18″-24″ length.
2. Make a loop at one end of the strip by folding over the terminal 3 inches of the strip onto itself and rubber cementing it together.
3. Place this loop over the 5th toe and direct the remaining length of the strip dorsally.
4. Exerting sufficient tension on the loop to bring the 5th toe into proper alignment, pass the rubber strip obliquely across the dorsal aspect of the foot, proximal to the head of the first metatarsal, down over the longitudinal arch, obliquely across the plantar aspect of the foot, proximally to the base of the fifth metatarsal, inferiorly to the lateral malleolus, around the posterior aspect of the heel, inferiorly to the medial malleolus, and distally to meet the strip that lies on the dorsomedial aspect of the foot.
5. Trim any excess length past the strip on the dorsum.
6. Remove the strip from the foot and adhere the terminal portion to the appropriate area of the strip that lies on the dorsum.
7. Trim a shallow U from the rubber loop that will lie in the interdigital web space.

Gibbard, L.C., *Charlesworth's Chiropodial Orthopedics*, London, Balliere, Tindall, and Cassell, 1968, p. 41.

TRACTION SLING FOR OVERLAPPING FIFTH TOE

INDICATIONS

To help correct the position of an overlapping 5th toe deformity.

MATERIALS

¾" to 1" wide strip rubber, rubber cement, scissors.

BOUNDARIES

The device is looped over the fifth digit, with a length of strip rubber passing obliquely across the plantar aspect of the foot (from distal lateral to proximal medial) and around the ankle.

CONSTRUCTION

1. Cut a ¾" to 1" wide strip of rubber to an 18"-24" length.
2. Make a loop at one end of the strip by folding over the terminal 3 inches of the strip onto itself and rubber cementing it together.
3. Place this loop over the 5th toe and direct the remaining length of the strip plantarly.
4. Exerting sufficient tension on the loop to bring the 5th toe into proper alignment, pass the rubber strip obliquely across the plantar aspect of the foot, proximal to the head of the first metatarsal, up over the longitudinal arch, laterally across the dorsum of the foot, inferiorly to the lateral malleolus, around the posterior aspect of the heel, and inferiorly to the medial malleolus thereby meeting the strip on the dorsomedial aspect of the foot.
5. Trim any excess length past the strip on the dorsum.
6. Remove the strip from the foot and adhere the terminal portion to the appropriate area of the strip that lies on the dorsum.
7. Trim a shallow U from the rubber strip that will lie in the interdigital web space.

Gibbard, L.C., *Charlesworth's Chiropodial Orthopedics*, London, Balliere, Tindall, and Cassell, 1968, p. 39.

IX
BIBLIOGRAPHY

Appel, Gustave. Protective Ballet Toe Pad. *Journal of the National Association of Chiropodists*, 44 (15): 1954, pp. 36-38.

Batts, Victor L., and P.E. Balloqui. The Technique of Latex Appliance Making. *The Chiropodist*, 5 (12): 1950, pp. 348-353.

Bell, W. Jackson. The Interference Pad. *Current Podiatry*, 15 (5): May 1966, p. 21.

Bellin, E.D. *The Practical Chiropodist*. London: The New Era Publishing Co. Ltd., pp. 145-157.

Berger, A.E. Padding with Textile Foot Covers. *Journal of the National Association of Chiropodists*, 31 (3): 1941, pp. 14-16.

Berger, O.R. Orthopedic Padding. *Chiropody Record*, 26 (7): 1943, pp. 135-139.

_____. Shoe Padding for Bunions and Melonia Dura. *Chiropody Record*, 28 (2): February 1945, pp. 17-20.

_____. Orthopedic Padding. *Chiropody Record*, 26 (4): 1943, pp. 72, 73, 84.

_____. Orthopedic Padding. *Chiropody Record*, 26 (5): 1943, pp. 87-90.

_____. Orthopedic Padding. *Chiropody Record*, 26 (6): 1943, pp. 111-113.

Blakely, D.L. Latex Toe Shield Made on Cast Taken Under Weight Pressure. *Clinical Journal of Chiropody and Podiatry*, 11 (2): 1940, pp. 52-54.

Block, Irving. Static Latex Shielding. *Current Chiropody*, 9: Sept. 1956, pp. 9-11.

Bluhm, Lester W. A New Technique for Rehabilitation of the Forefoot. *Journal of the National Association of Chiropodists*, 41 (6): 1951.

Blum, David. A New Dressing for Routine Palliative Work. *Journal of the National Association of Chiropodists*, 45 (10): 1955, p. 53.

Bradley, J. Bennett. Shielding. *Chiropody Review*, 6 (3): March 1945, p. 39.

Brookes, Denis. The Second Toe and Hallux Valgus. *The Chiropodist*, 24 (209): 1937, pp. 275-276.

Burkhead, Harold R. Diagnosis and Treatment of Forefoot Conditions. *British Journal of Chiropodists*, 21 (4): 1956, pp. 82-85, 91-92.

Burnett, Edwin K. *M.J. Lewi Textbook of Chiropody*. New York: School of Chiropody of New York, 1914, pp. 909-949.

Burnett, Gross. *Practice of Podiatry*, pp. 81-126.

Challoner, Alan. The Theory of Padding and Strapping. *British Journal of Chiropody*, 29 (7): 1964, pp. 169-171.

Charlesworth, Franklin. *Chiropody—Theory and Practice*, 1961, pp. 478-518.

_____. Combine Met. Pad with Toe Loop and Heel Loop. *British Journal of Chiropody*, 23 (10): 1958, pp. 272-273.

_____. Simple Pad and Brace Techniques. *British Journal of Chiropody*, 24 (1): 1959, pp. 10-13.

Coates, I.S. Animal Wool Technique. *British Journal of Chiropody*, 37 (6): 1972, pp. 133, 156.

_____. Chairside Replaceable Plantar Toe Props. *The Chiropodist*, 23: 1968, pp. 316-318.

_____. Practical Appliances. *The Chiropodist*, 19 (7): July 1964, pp. 169-171.

_____. Silicone Rubber Foot Devices. *British Journal of Chiropody*, 37 (11): 1972, pp. 245-246.

_____. Silicone Rubber Foot Devices (Part 3). *British Journal of Chiropody*, 37 (11): 1972, pp. 273-275.

_____. Silicone Rubber Foot Devices (Part 9). *British Journal of Chiropody*, 38 (6): 1973, pp. 125-127.

Connolly, Thomas F. Thermoplastics and Plantar Lesions. *Current Podiatry*, 17 (3): 1966, pp. 9-11.

Davis, A. A Removable Bunion Pad. *Chiropody Review*, 12 (3): March 1951, pp. 57-60.

_____. A Removable Toe Prop. *Chiropody Review*, 12 (1): 1951, pp. 5-7.

Dietz, Lorraine H. Perforated Latex Appliances. *Clinical Journal of Chiropody, Podiatry and Pedic Surgery*, 12 (2): 1941, p. 63.

Dowdeswell-Childs, T.G. Replaceable Padding for Geriatrics Patient. *The Chiropodist*, 21 (1): Jan. 1966, pp. 4-7.

_____. Replaceable Padding for Geriatrics. *The Chiropodist*, 21 (1): Jan. 1966, pp. 33-37.

Drew, F.A. *Latex Telchnique and Its Application to Chiropody*. London: The Actinic Press, 1951.

_____. Removable Padding. *British Journal of Chiropody*, 20 (1): 1955, pp. 13-17.

_____. Removable Padding. *Current Chiropody*, 8: October 1955, pp. 9-13.

Drummer, Benjamin. A Departure in Padding for Metarsalgia. *Journal of National Association of Chiropodists*, 35 (18): 1945.

Ellison, William E. Toe Flex Pad. *Current Chiropody*, 6 (5): 1952, pp. 9-11.

Endersby, M.E. Removable Hallaux Valgus Pad. *Chiropodist*, 4 (3): 1949, pp. 66-67.

Fisher, Carlman. A New Technique in Orthodigital Correction. *Journal of American Podiatry Association*, 53 (3): March 1963, pp. 187-191.

Ford, H.P. and A.W. Swallow. An Appliance for the Extensor Tendon of Great Toe. *The Chiropodist*, 10 (8): 1955, pp. 248-250.

Gibbard, Laurence C. *Charlesworth's Chiropodial Orthopedics*. London: Balliere, Tindall and Cassell, 1968, pp. 37-64.

_____. Plantar Padding, Part I. *British Journal of Chiropody*, 23 (7): 1958, p. 178.

_____. Plantar Padding, Part II. *British Journal of Chiropody*, 23 (8): 1958, pp. 203-204.

_____. The Management and Treatment of Digital Hard Corns. *British Journal of Chiropody*, 23 (10): 1957, pp. 247-252.

_____. Padding the Met. Heads. *British Journal of Chiropody*, 21 (1): 1956, pp. 188-191.

Guidice, Robert A. Dynamic Balance Therapy. *Current Podiatry*, 11 (2): Feb. 1962, pp. 16-17.

Gorick, Gillian M. Trial of Sheepskin Boots in the Prevention of Pressure Areas on the Feet. *Chiropodist* (from *New Zealand Journal of Physiotherapy*), Oct. 1969, pp. 381-385.

Hanby, John H. *Principles of Chiropody*. London: Balliere, Tindall and Cox, pp. 124-146.

Hawes, K. Duncan. Leather Padding. *Chiropodist*, 18 (12): Dec. 1963, pp. 361-364.

Healy, Frank. Rubber Sponge—Its Use in Chiropody. *Chiropody Record*, 17 (5): 1934, p. 119.

Hymes, Leonard. Corrections for Focal Point of Pressure. *Current Podiatry*, 12 (11): Nov. 1963, pp. 7-19.

_____. A Toe Aligning Sling. *Current Podiatry*, 14 (7): 1965, pp. 7-11.

Jardine, K. Lewis. An Alternative Approach to Sustained Plantar Pads. *Chiropodist*, 17 (10): Oct. 1962, pp. 283-284.

Jones, Keith Campbell. *The Practice of Chiropody*. London: Angus and Robertson, 1948, pp. 245-252.

Jones, Ted. A Technique for Dynamically Molding Shields and Orthodigital Devices. *Current Podiatry*, 16 (6): June 1967, pp. 7-9.

Joseph, Alfred. An Ideal Bunion Shield. *Chiropody Record*, 8 (9): 1925, p. 12.

_____. *Practical Podiatry*. New York: First Institute of Podiatry, 1918, pp. 96-142.

_____. Treatment of Common Corn. *Chiropody Record*, 8 (9): p. 5.

Kaegi, George A. Proper Cast—Proper Appliance. *The Chiropody Review*, 15 (5): May 1954, pp. 21-22.

Karr, Joseph. Method to Alleviate and Cure Painful Heel Syndrome. *JAPA*, 68 (2): Feb. 1978, pp. 124-126.

Knapp, Janice C. Orthopedic Strappings. *Clinical Journal of Chiropody*, 11 (2): 1940, p. 55.

Koehler, Paul O. Bunion Casting and Padding. *Journal of the National Association of Chiropodists*, 25 (11): 1935, pp. 10-11.

_____. Toe Casting Board. *Clinical Journal of Chiropody, Podiatry and Pedic Surgery*, 10 (10): 1934, pp. 333-334.

Koppe, W.P. Palliative Padding and Strapping. *Clinical Journal of Chiropody*, 5 (6): 1933, pp. 184-187.

_____. Palliative Padding and Stripping. *Clinical Journal of Chiropody*, 5 (7): 1933, pp. 229-231.

_____. Palliative Padding and Strapping. *Clinical Journal of Chiropody*, 5 (10): 1933, pp. 329-331.

_____. Palliative Padding and Strapping. *Clinical Journal of Chiropody*, 5 (12): 1933, pp. 426-427.

_____. Palliative Padding and Strapping. *Clinical Journal of Chiropody*, 6 (1): 1934, pp. 7-8.

_____. Palliative Padding and Strapping. *Clinical Journal of Chiropody*, 6 (2): 1934, pp. 43, 45, 55.

_____. Palliative Padding and Strapping. *Clinical Journal of Chiropody*, 6 (4): 1934, pp. 118-119, 124.

_____. Palliative Padding and Strapping. *Clinical Journal of Chiropody*, 6 (5): 1934, pp. 155-158.

Krout, Robert R. A Common Source of Foot Symptomatology (1). *Current Podiatry*, 10 (9): Sept. 1961, pp. 9-14.

_____. A Common Source of Foot Symptomatology (2). *Current Podiatry*, 10 (10): 1961, pp. 17-19.

_____. A Common Source of Foot Symptomatology (3). *Current Podiatry*, 10 (11): Nov. 1961, pp. 18-23.

_____. Do Standard Paddings Improve Foot Function Adequately. *Current Podiatry*, 12 (9): Sept. 1963, pp. 14-17.

_____. Shock Absorbing Pads for Symptomatic Feet. *Current Podiatry*, 24: Dec. 1975, pp. 8-12.

Lancet, David. The Self-Moulded Felt Balancer. *Current Chiropody*, 12 (6): June 1955, pp. 12, 16.

Larson, Alvin C. Podiatric Use of a Premedicated Pad. *J.A.P.A.*, 52 (3): March 1962, p. 206.

Lederman, Erwin S. Toe Corrector. *Chiropody Record*, 26 (12): 1943, pp. 227-231.

Leydecker, Chas. P., and W.C. Cartledge. Shielding the Little Toe. *Chiropody Record*, 17: 1934, pp. 175-177.

Lombard, Herman, Kolika. A New Material in Podiatry. *Current Podiatry*, 21: November 1972, p. 19.

Mann, Roger A. *DuVries Surgery of the Foot*. St. Louis: C.V. Mosby Co., 1973, pp. 425-435.

McDonald, R. Hand Moulded Plastizote Appliances. *The Chiropodist*, 22: July 1967, pp. 235-239.

Meldman, E.C. The Improved Latex Technique. *Chiropody Record*, 23 (5): May 1940, pp. 91-93.

_____. The Improved Latex Technique. *Chiropody Record*, 23: 1940, pp. 11-12.

_____. The Improved Latex Technique. *Chiropody Record*, 23 (7): July 1940, pp. 151-153, 158-163.

_____. Review of Casting Methods for Latex Appliances. *Chiropody Record*, 20 (1): 1937, p. 6.

Mennel, James. Some Disabilities of the Foot and Their Treatment. *The Chiropodist*, 22 (181): May 1935, pp. 178-181.

Mercante, Ralph P. Acrylic Toe Spreader for the Interdigital Lesion. *Current Podiatry*, 18 (17): 1969, pp. 7-9.

Michaels, Charles A. A Chairside Appliance Material. *Current Podiatry*, 18 (5): May 1969, pp. 20-21.

_____. Use of Polyfoam in Podiatry. *Current Podiatry*, 9: June 1960, pp. 18-19.

Moccia, Arthur A. Suggestions in Shielding. *Current Podiatry*, 4: April 1955, p. 14.

Moon, Cecil L. Principles and Practice of Latex Therapy. *Current Chiropody*, 11: Nov. 1953, pp. 9-11.

O'Connell, John F. A New Method for Adhering Felt Paddings. *Chiropody Record*, 30 (12): 1937, pp. 323-324.

_____. Padding. *Chiropody Record*, 14 (3): 1931, pp. 7-13.

Parker, O.C. How Do You Treat Soft Corns? *Chiropody Record*, 8 (4): 1925, p. 17.

Pasternack, A.B. An Ingenious Pad. *Chiropody Record*, 17 (7): 1934, pp. 180-181.

_____. Electrical Pads. *Chiropody Record*, 18 (11): 1935, pp. 274-276.

_____. Pads and Plasters. *Chiropody Record*, 17 (2): 1934, pp. 45-46.

Polokoff, Morton M. A Buttress Appliance to Extend 2nd, 3rd and 4th Toes. *J.A.P.A.*, 64 (10): 1974, pp. 798-803.

_____. A Latex Bunion Shield Which Can Be Adjusted to Protect Secondary Lesions. *J.A.P.A.*, 65 (3): March 1975, pp. 250-257.

_____. A Treatment for Morton's Neuralgia. *Journal of National Association of Chiropodists*, 38 (5): 1948, pp. 27-31.

_____. Contracted Fourth Toe Traction Appliance. *J.A.P.A.*, 65 (11): 1975, pp. 1074-1075.

_____. Double Ring Felt Appliance to Provide Traction for Dorsally Contracted Second Toe. *J.A.P.A.*, 65 (1): 1975, pp. 60-65.

_____. Felt Pads for the Bunion Joints 1st and 5th. *Current Chiropody*, 11: Feb. 1954, pp. 11-12.

_____. Lesser Toe Latex Shield Made with Tubular Gauze. *J.A.P.A.*, 48 (9): 1958, pp. 432-433.

_____. Orthodigita: Removable Felt and Silicone Appliances for Conservative Treatment of Hypermobility of the First Segment. *J.A.P.A.*, 64 (9): Sept. 1974, pp. 721-729.

_____. Orthodigital Traction Appliance to Correct Heloma Durum on 5th Toe. *Journal of the National Association of Chiropodists*, 36 (1): 1946, pp. 7-9.

_____. Orthodigita Treatment. *Australian Podiatrist*, 9 (4): Nov. 1975.

_____. Polokoff Buttress Appliance. *Chiropody Record*, 39 (1-2): 1956, pp. 6-8.

_____. The Polokoff Hallux Shield. *J.A.P.A.*, 60 (12): Dec. 1970, pp. 480-483.

_____. The Polokoff Pad. *Journal of the National Association of Chiropodists*, 35 (12): 1945, pp. 16-18.

_____. Removable Appliances to Protect Deformities on the Same Foot. *Australian Podiatrist*, 10 (1): Feb. 1976, pp. 74-79.

_____. Removable Bunion Appliance. *Journal of the National Association of Chiropodists*, 36 (9): 1946, pp. 18-19.

_____. Removable Felt Appliances to Protect Multiple Deformities on the Same Foot. *J.A.P.A.*, 64 (11): Nov. 1974, pp. 890-898.

_____. Removable Shield for Lesions About Head of 5th Metatarsal. *J.A.P.A.*, 57 (12): 1967, pp. 556-558.

_____. A Simplified Casting Technique. *Clinical Journal of Chiropody, Podiatry and Pedic Surgery*, 10 (6): 1939, pp. 189-191.

_____. Specialized Pad for Overlapping Second Toes. *Current Podiatry*, 1953, p. 16.

_____. Traction Appliance for Third Toe. *J.A.P.A.*, 65 (10): 1975, pp. 1011-1012.

Raff, Joseph. Cynamic Foot Mold with Ant. Metatarsophalasq. Crest. *Current Chiropody*, May 1952, pp. 17-19.

Reese, Mose. A Buttress Appliance for Contracted Toes. *Journal of the National Association of Chiropodists*, 47 (1): 1957, pp. 18-19.

Rhymer, Ronald F. An Accurate Method of Toe Casting. *Current Podiatry*, 10 (4): 1961, pp. 23-24.

Rice, E.C. Shielding and Dressing. *Journal of National Association of Chiropodists*, 22 (11): 1932, pp. 18-19.

Rosenstein, Henry. Construction of a Permanent and Hygienic Met. Pad. *The Chiropodist*, 3 (2): Feb. 1948.

Rosoff, Samuel. The Fabrication of Orthotic Devices with the Use of Silicone Gel. *J.A.P.A.*, 60 (8): Aug. 1970, pp. 313-321.

Roven, Milton D. A Latex Forefoot Device with Threefold Action. *J.A.P.A.*, 48 (9): Sept. 1958, pp. 417-418.

Runting, E.G.V. The Ageing Foot. *The Chiropodist*, 27 (241): May 1940, pp. 125-131.

_____. *Practical Chiropody*. St. Louis: The C.V. Mosby Co., 1929, pp. 100-125.

Sansone, Ralph E. Parallel Strip Padding for Weight Stress Distribution and Redirection. *J.A.P.A.*, 60 (5): May 1970, pp. 193-198.

Schneider, Lawrence W. A Simplified Removable Corn Shield. *Journal of the National Association of Chiropodists*, 39 (11): 1949, pp. 35-37.

Schuster, Otto. *Foot Orthopedics*. 1927, pp. 286-288.

Schuster, R.O. The C. Mold. *Current Chiropody*, Jan. 1956, pp. 13-14.

Sherman, L.H. An Original Method for Making an Inlay. *Journal New Jersey Chiropodists Society*, April 1952, pp. 13, 14.

Silverman, J.J. Dynamic-State Orthodigital Appliances. *Current Podiatry*, 12 (10): Oct. 1963, pp. 7, 8, 11, 12, 14.

Silverman, Leonard F., and Herman G. Pollack. Shielding of Orthodigital Devices with Rubber Silicones. *J.A.P.A.*, March 1962, p. 205.

Simko, Michael V. Economy in Padding. *Chiropody Record*, 38 (7-8): p. 27.

_____. Presenting Gauze. *Chiropody Record*, 1928, p. 3.

Sivitz, Sidney C. A New Resilient Plastic for Orthodigital Prosthetics. *Journal of National Association of Chiropodists*, 47 (4): April 1957, pp. 172-175.

_____. Technique for Fabricating Toe Shields. *Journal of the National Association of Chiropodists*, 43 (3): 1953, pp. 32-37.

Smith, Hal P. Revised Method of Making Bunion Shields with Rubber Butter and Liquid Rubber. *Chiropody Record*, 19 (6): 1936, p. 163.

Snuff, E.B. A Latex Appliance for Heloma Molle. *Chiropody Record*, p. 3.

Solomon, Gilbert. Casting of the Toe for Latex Shield Without Separating Medium. *Current Chiropody*, Oct. 1959, pp. 5, 6.

Solomon, Sanford E. The Practicality and Economy of Felt. *Chiropody Record*, 18 (7): 1935, pp. 173-175.

Sonderling, Herman. *Gross's Modern Foot Therapy*, pp. 518-626.

Stern, Arthur L. A New Method for Latex Plantar Appliances. *Current Chiropody*, Dec. 1954, pp. 13-14.

Stern, William. The True Dynamic Appliance. *Current Chiropody*, May 1953, pp. 17-19.

Stillman, E.G. A Simple Dynamic Foot Mold. *Current Podiatry*, July 1960, pp. 9-10.

Stirling, R. The Cutting Out of Pads. *The Chiropodist*, 5 (6): 1950, pp. 167-169.

Stone, Jack. Therapeutic Padding for Heloma Molle. *Current Podiatry*, 16 (1): 1967, pp. 18-19.

Strans, Raymond. Plastic Rubber Appliances. *Clinical Journal of Chiropodists, Podiatrists and Pedic Surgery*, 11 (2): 1940, pp. 54-55.

Sturtz, Harry. Dynamic Foot Mould Therapy. *Current Chiropody*, Feb. 1952, pp. 6-8.

Trill, Henry. *Corns and Callosities in the 4th Cleft*. London: Actinic Press, 1951, pp. 44-47.

Turvey, Jesse W.J. Digital Appliances by the Coagulant Salt Process. *The Chiropodist*, 11 (9): Sept. 1956, pp. 267-269.

Unknown. Jottings. *The Chiropodist*, 21 (171): July 1934, pp. 211-214.

Unknown. A New Way of Staying on Your Toes. *British Journal of Chiropody*, 38 (8): 1973, p. 179.

Van Hes, Bel. Some Aspects of Palliative Treatment in Chiropody. *Chiropody Review*, 7 (4): April 1946, pp. 70-72.

Vosburg, G.B. Liquid Latex Technique. *Clinical Journal of Chiropody, Podiatry and Pedic Surgery*, 9 (7): 1937, pp. 249-253.

_____. Palliative for Hallux Valgus. *Clinical Journal of Chiropody, Podiatry and Pedic Surgery*, 3 (7): 1930, pp. 219-220.

Walker, H.E. An Aspect of Padding. *The Chiropodist*, 13 (7): July 1958, pp. 198-199.

_____. Some Fallacies in the Theory of Padding. *The Chiropodist*, 25 (218): June 1938, pp. 185-187.

Walker, Morton, and Eric J. Rothstein. Adjunctive Therapy for Plantar Lesions. *Current Podiatry*, p. 10.

Walker, Morton H. Crest Appliance for Dispensing. *Current Podiatry*, 11 (17): July 1962, pp. 19-20.

_____. A Protective Foot Guard. *Current Podiatry*, 10 (9): Sept. 1961, pp. 25-26.

Wardle, Arthur. Essentials in the Technique of Padding and Strapping.

Warmbath, H. Fallacies in the Theory of Padding. *The Chiropodist*, 25 (219): July 1938, pp. 229-230.

Watts, W.D. Chairside Appliances. *Current Podiatry*, 17 (2): Feb. 1968, pp. 7-10.

_____. Detachable and Replaceable Dressings. *British Journal of Chiropody*, 1957, pp. 303-305.

_____. Padding—A Comparison. *British Journal of Chiropody*, 20 (6): 1955, pp. 148-149.

Weinstein, Frank. *Principles and Practice of Podiatry*. Philadelphia: Lea and Febiger, 1968, pp. 264-276.

Whitney, Alan K. Orthodigital Control of Underlapping 5th Toe. *Current Podiatry*, 13 (12): Dec. 1964, pp. 20-22.

_____. *Urethane Mold Therapy, Study Packet*. Philadelphia: PCPM, 1971.

_____. Urethane Moulding. *British Journal of Chiropody*, 33 (1): 1968, pp. 22.

Woolf, William. *Toe Casting and Liquid Rubber Technic*. New York: Harriman Printing Co., 1937, pp. 49-88.

Wright, F. Bennett. Balanced Casting. *Current Chiropody*, Nov. 1952, pp. 13, 14, 16.

Yale, Irving. *Podiatric Medicine*. Baltimore: Williams and Wilkins Co., 1974, pp. 16-17, 252-265.

_____. *Podiatric Medicine*. Baltimore: Williams and Wilkins Co., 1974, pp. 98-102.

_____. *Podiatric Medicine*. Baltimore: Williams and Wilkins Co., pp. 119-122.